THE MEDITERRANEAN DIET COOKBOOK FOR BEGINNERS

5 WEEK PLANS AND 160 QUICK & EASY MEDITERRANEAN RECIPES
FOR
CLEAN & HEALTHY LIFE, FROM BREAKFAST TO DINNER

Amber Hultin

© Copyright 2022 - All rights reserved.

The content contained within this book may not be reproduced, duplicated or transmitted without direct written permission from the author or the publisher. Under no circumstances will any blame or legal responsibility be held against the publisher, or author, for any damages, reparation, or monetary loss due to the information contained within this book. Either directly or indirectly.

Legal Notice:

This book is copyright protected. This book is only for personal use. You cannot amend, distribute, sell, use, quote or paraphrase any part, or the content within this book, without the consent of the author or publisher.

Disclaimer Notice:

Please note the information contained within this document is for educational and entertainment purposes only. All effort has been executed to present accurate, up to date, and reliable, complete information. No warranties of any kind are declared or implied. Readers acknowledge that the author is not engaging in the rendering of legal, financial, medical or professional advice. The content within this book has been derived from various sources. Please consult a licensed professional before attempting any techniques outlined in this book.

By reading this document, the reader agrees that under no circumstances is the author responsible for any losses, direct or indirect, which are incurred as a result of the use of information contained within this document, including, but not limited to, errors, omissions, or inaccuracies.

TABLE OF CONTENTS

INTRODUCTION 10

CHAPTER 1 16

LOW GI DIETS AND ITS IMPORTANCE 16

CHAPTER 2 20

MEDITERRANEAN DIET 20

CHAPTER 3 22

GLYCEMIC INDEX OF MAIN FOODS 22

CHAPTER 4 26

MEAL PLAN 26

    5 WEEKS MEAL PLAN 29

CHAPTER 5 34

BREAKFAST 34

    RECIPES 35

        Mediterranean Pita With Chicken, Bell Pepper Andra, mean Roasted Garlic 35

        Toast With Roasted Tomatoes And Crushed Avocado 36

        Roasted Almond Honey Bars 36

        Chickpea And Spinach Stew 37

        Main ingredients 37

        German Pancakes Recipe 37

        Lebanese Cheese Fatayers 38

        Vegan Pesto Manchego Empanada 38

        Blackberry, Banana And Yogurt Popsicles 40

- Spanish Toast 40
- Tangerine, Cocoa And Evoo Muffins 41
- Labneh With Garlic And Mint 42
- Vegan Chickpea And Chocolate Cookies 42
- Muhammara 42
- Mallorcan Empanadas 43
- Tahini 44
- Artichoke And Spinach Frittata 44
- Balsamic Berries With Honey Yogurt 45
- Avocado Caprese Toast 45
- Spinach And Feta Breakfast Roll 45
- Easy Muesli 46
- Egg Toast With Lemon Yogurt 46
- Mediterranean Breakfast With Pita Bread 46
- Oatmeal Smoothie 47
- Bean Salad With Avocado And Quinoa 47
- Bread With Tomato, Oil, And Garlic 47
- Mediterranean Salad 48
- Banana Nut Muffins 100% Whole Grain 48
- Hummus 49
- Pita With Eggs And Vegetables 49
- Egg And Mushrooms On Toast 49
- Baked Eggs 50
- Chickpea Egg Bowl 50
- Fresh Cheese with Tomato 51
- Broccoli & Eggs 51
- Garlic Eggs 51
- Banana Quinoa 52
- Almond Risotto 52
- Coconut Risotto 52
- Breakfast Quinoa 52

Coconut Yogurt 53

Squash & Apple Porridge 53

Refreshing Mango and Pear Smoothie 53

Barley Porridge 54

Strawberry and Rhubarb Smoothie 54

Cheesy Zucchini Omelette 54

Easy to Munch Olive Cherry and Olive Bites 55

Power Packed Oatmeal 55

Banana Steel Oats 55

Hearty Pumpkin Oats 55

Cool Red Pepper and Olive Omelette 56

Avocado and Blueberry Medley 56

CHAPTER 6 58

LUNCH 58

RECIPES 60

Hot Spinach And Artichoke Cups 60

Salad With Chickpeas, Bulgur, And Orange 60

Bruschetta With Balsamic Dressing, Olives, And Pepper 61

Mediterranean Marinated Vegetable Salad 61

Mediterranean Cheese 62

Zucchini And Aubergines Stuffed With Tomato And Cheese 62

Shrimp Bruschetta With Orzo Pasta 62

Caesar Salad With Romaine Lettuce And 63

Grilled Chicken 63

Spanish paella 63

Grilled Chicken With Fresh Spinach And Tomato Confit 64

Chicken With Spinach And Lemon Cream 65

Chicken Breast With Fennel Salad 66

Grilled Chicken With Chanterelles And Pumpkin 66

Chicken With Tomato Compote And Cornicabra 67

Chicken Breast With Parsnip And Rosemary Sauce 68

Grilled Chicken With Bimi, Soy Sauce And Kimchi 68

Chicken Stuffed With Kale And Toum Sauce 69

Chicken With Lemon And Hot Spices 70

Chicken Breast With Boletus And Spinach 70

Chicken Skewers With Satay Sauce 71

Aubergine Flatbread With Roasted Garlic And Sepionets 72

Cuttlefish With Ginger And Coconut Milk 73

Asparagus Skewer And Cuttlefish Carpaccio With Parmesan 73

Cuttlefish Skewers With Romesco Sauce 74

Sautéed Chickpeas With Cuttlefish 75

Cuttlefish Casserole With Mushrooms 75

Cuttlefish With Pickled Courgette 76

Cuttlefish Tagine With Lemon 76

Italian Chicken 77

Turkey Verde with Brown Rice 77

Turkey Meatloaf 78

Turkey Lasagna 78

Eggplant Salad 78

Tender Watermelon and Radish Salad 79

Tasty Yogurt and Cucumber Salad 79

Herbed Up Feisty Baby Potatoes 79

Mesmerizing Brussels and Pistachios 79

Fancy Greek Orzo Salad 80

Cheesy Roasted Broccoli 80

Mediterranean Kale Dish 80

Shrimp in White Wine 81

CHAPTER 7 82

DINNER 82

Recipes 82

Title	Page
Pumpkin Cream Recipe With Trumpet Of Death, Cheese Crumbs, And Confit Garlic Cream	82
Pumpkin And Clove Cream With Kale Sprouts	83
Roasted Pumpkin Cream With Sage	84
Pumpkin Cream With Roasted Chickpeas And Avocado	84
Pumpkin Cream With Light Escarole And Parmesan Stew	85
Pumpkin Cream, Ham And Pine Nuts	86
Pumpkin And Coconut Cream	87
Pumpkin Cream With Smoked Herring Roe And Black Garlic	88
Pumpkin And Turnip Cream	88
Pumpkin Cream With Mi Cuit Foie And Black Truffle	89
Chickpea And Pumpkin Hummus	90
Pumpkin Gazpacho	90
Hake With Tomatoes Marinated In Soy	91
Baked Bream With Arugula And Ham	92
Grilled Sea Bream With Clams	92
Low-Temperature Teriyaki Cod	93
Salmon With Broccoli And Almond Cream	94
Salmon With Sesame And Orange, A Delicious And Easy Recipe For Air Fryer	95
Baked Sea Bass With Oyster Mushrooms And Pickled Lemon	95
Baked Sea Bass With Potatoes And Spring Garlic	96
Mullets With Red Cabbage With Ginger And Sesame	97
Salad Of Verdinas, Prawns, And Spinach	97
Mediterranean Boneless	98
Lentil, Smoked Salmon And Avocado Salad	99
Bean Salad With Avocado, Tomato And Sweet And Sour Radishes	99
Tasty Beef and Broccoli	100
Beef Corn Chili	100
Balsamic Beef Dish	101
Soy Sauce Beef Roast	101
Rosemary Beef Chuck Roast	102
Pork Chops and Tomato Sauce	102

- Pork Potato 102
- Pasta Carbonara 103
- Margherita Pizza 103
- Mushroom Risotto 104
- Pasta Con Pomodoro E Basilico 105
- Fettuccine Pomodoro 105
- Classic Pasta Amatriciana 106

CHAPTER 8 108

SNACKS AND SIDES 108

RECIPES 108

- Tomato, Avocado, Egg And Sweet And Sour Cucumber Sandwich ... 108
- White Bean And Bacon Dip 108
- Avocado, Mozzarella, And Roasted Pepper 109
- Pate Sandwich 109
- Ham And Brie Cheese Piadina 109
- Crispy And Spicy Chickpeas 110
- Carrot Chips 110
- Cherry-Peach Compote with Greek Yogurt 111
- Roasted Peach and Orange Crostini 111
- Pumpkin Yogurt Parfait 112
- Chocolate-Coated Dates 112
- Cashew and Peanut Rice Pudding 113
- Apple Crisp 113
- White Bean Dip 113
- Grilled Flatbread with Burrata Cheese 114
- Fruicuterie Board 114
- Baked Beet Chips 115
- Smoked Salmon and Avocado Summer Rolls 115
- Grab-and-Go Snack Jars 116
- Blueberry Coconut Energy Bites 116

All-Green Crudités Basket 117

Falafel Smash 117

Healthy Lemon Bars 118

Beet Hummus 118

Roasted Veggie Chips 119

Rainbow Heirloom Tomato Bruschetta 119

Fava Bean Guacamole With Root Chips 120

Roasted Pepper And Eggplant Spread Recipe 121

Pumpkin Hummus 122

Triple-Berry Smoothie Bowl 122

Vegan Brownie Bites 123

Crispy BBQ Roasted Chickpeas 123

Veggie Sushi 124

CONCLUSIONS 126

Introduction

Having a balanced diet is essential to combat overweight and obesity, and other pathologies increasingly have an increasing incidence in today's society. It is not about following a strict and restrictive diet but about providing the body with all the necessary nutrients to carry out its vital functions.

Do you know the etymology of the word "diet"? It is very revealing since it comes from the Greek diatia (δίαιτα), which means "way of life." And it is that how we feed ourselves constitutes a habit and, therefore, a way of living.
Although the word diet is often used -in an erroneous way- to refer to restrictive regimens aimed at losing weight or linked to some disease, the diet is, in reality, the set of foods, their quantity, and frequency with which they are eaten, Which are ingested.
In the case of human beings, food is conditioned by cultural, geographical, climatic, economic, and social factors and, in addition, by individual tastes.

Differences Between Food, Nutrition, And Dietetics

The terms food, nutrition, and dietetics are sometimes used interchangeably, but you should know that they are not the same:
Food refers to the entire process by which we supply our body with food; this process is essential for living beings to obtain energy. It encompasses both the preparation or cooking of food and its intake. It varies according to individual and social circumstances.
Nutrition refers to how the body transforms the ingested food, incorporating its nutrients into the body.
Dietetics is a discipline linked to food and nutrition, which studies the most appropriate foods and feeding methods according to individual circumstances, such as age, sex, or the presence of pathologies to maintain health.
As we have seen, nutrients are part of the food we eat in the feeding process.
An adequate diet, which provides the body with the nutrients it needs, combined with regular physical activity, is the key to good health. On the contrary, a poor diet can negatively affect the immune system's capacity and subtract physical and mental energy to carry out basic activities normally.
Human beings need six main groups of nutrients divided into two categories based on the amount needed:

•	Macronutrients: we need them in a greater quantity, and their fundamental role is energy contribution.

•	Carbohydrates (or carbohydrates, carbohydrates, or hydrates): they serve to provide our body with the energy necessary to function.
They can be of two kinds:

1.	Simple: they break down quickly and therefore provide energy quickly. For example, honey, sugar, or white rice.

2.	Complex: They break down more slowly, releasing energy more slowly. For example, pasta or whole wheat bread.

While its excessive intake can lead to diseases such as obesity or diabetes, its deficiency can result in fatigue or weakening of muscle tissue (as the body is forced to obtain energy from protein).

Proteins: they are made up of amino acids, and in addition to providing energy, they have a structural function since they are involved in the formation of muscle tissue, enzymes, hormones, antibodies, etc. When there is a lack of these, health problems such as loss of muscle mass can occur.
There are nine essential amino acids (valine, leucine, isoleucine, threonine, lysine, methionine, histidine, phenylalanine, tryptophan), which the body cannot synthesize and are essential for creating proteins, so they must be supplied through the diet. Proteins can be found in meat, fish, eggs, dairy products, legumes, and seafood.

Lipids (or fats) play an important role in our body; they mainly do not provide energy, transport fat-soluble vitamins, and are a structural part of cell membranes.
We distinguish two types:

•	Saturated fats: structurally, they do not contain double bonds (unsaturation), hence their name. They are usually solid at room temperature and come from animal or vegetable oils, such as coconut or palm oil. They are not considered healthy fats, and their consumption should be limited.

•	Unsaturated fats: structurally, they have at least one double bond. They are liquid at room temperature and found in oils such as olive or sunflower. They are divided into monounsaturated and polyunsaturated fats based on the number of double bonds they contain. These types of links modify the properties of lipids, so these fats are considered healthier. This group contains Omega-3 fatty acids, necessary for proper brain development, anti-inflammatory, and protection against cardiovascular events.

Lipids are necessary for the body to provide energy and protect vital organs. However, they should be ingested in moderation since excessive consumption leads to increased cholesterol and obesity, among other pathologies.

Micronutrients: they are necessary for very small quantities, but they are key for the proper functioning of the body. They usually have a repairing or plastic or regulatory function of certain cellular chemical reactions.
Vitamins are involved in many biological processes and are found in animal and vegetable origin foods, although the main source is fruits and vegetables. Each vitamin has specific functions. For example, vitamin C has an antioxidant effect, protecting the body from oxidative stress, A is also an antioxidant and has a key role in vision, and K is involved in blood coagulation. It is important to include a wide variety of fruits and vegetables and foods in general in the diet. In this way, we incorporate all the vitamins into our bodies.

Minerals: they are also essential for many processes in the body. Both its absence and excess generate various pathologies depending on the mineral. For example, a lack of calcium can cause osteoporosis, while an excess of sodium can cause hypertension.
Water: Although it is not strictly considered a nutrient, we include it in this category, given the importance of its daily intake. It has a fundamental role in the elimination of waste or digestion. We can provide it directly or through other products.
The importance of fiber

Fiber deserves a separate mention since, although it does not enter the group of nutrients because it cannot be digested, it contributes to important functions such as gastrointestinal transit, water absorption, cholesterol elimination, or glucose reduction, In blood and the level of fatty acids. In addition, it constitutes the food of the microbiota or intestinal flora, which is a set of microorganisms found in our intestine. The microbiota plays a very important role in health, but we are beginning to discover the extent of its importance today. We can highlight its participation in the immune system and digestive function among its functions. It is necessary to include fiber in our diet through fruits, vegetables, and whole grains for all these reasons.

The consequences of a lack of fiber can lead to diverticular disease of the colon, hemorrhoids, hiatal hernia, or varicose veins. By consuming foods rich in fiber, you will contribute to the prevention of all these pathologies, and, in addition, your cholesterol and risk of heart disease will be reduced.

A balanced diet is one in which foods from all the groups that we have seen are consumed, and that covers the recommended amounts of intake of each nutrient to guarantee the correct functioning of the organism.

The 6 Pillars Of A Balanced Diet

These are the six pillars on which a balanced diet is based:

1. Adapted: it must be personalized to the particularities of each person, their schedules, physical activity, economic conditions, age, health, etc.
2. Complete: it must provide all the nutrients, fiber, and water that our body needs in the right amounts.
3. Satisfactory: the food, the quantities, and the preparations must be appropriate and pleasant to feel satisfied; eating well does not have to be boring.
4. Varied: to get away from the monotony, it is advisable to vary our range of foods, in this way we ensure the contribution of all the minerals and vitamins. In addition, we must ensure that they are fresh and seasonal.
5. Balanced in energy: the energy contribution must be what we need; it is important for the correct functioning of our body not to overdo it or fall short.
6. Safe: it should not put our health at risk, preventing food poisoning and avoiding the intake of harmful components, such as fruit and vegetable pesticides or the abuse of additives.

As popular wisdom says, "we are what we eat." Indeed, food and health are closely linked. Numerous scientific studies support this. Recently an article in the prestigious magazine The Lancet exposed how "eating badly causes more deaths per year than tobacco." In his study on nutrition and health, he showed how the consumption of unhealthy foods leads to a significant increase in serious health problems.

In addition to those exposed in this study, a poor diet can also cause other problems such as for overweight and obesity, the latter classified by the WHO as a pandemic within non-infectious pathologies.

Diet is one of the most powerful tools to prevent diseases, so we must strive to make it balanced. We provide our body with all the necessary nutrients and properly perform all our biological functions in the right measure. In addition, we reduce the risk of suffering pathologies in the short, medium, and long term related to inadequate nutrition: hypertension, diabetes, obesity, cardiovascular diseases, even certain types of cancer, etc. The commitment to a balanced diet is the best health insurance we can buy ourselves.

As you have seen, the benefits of a balanced diet, always combined with a healthy lifestyle, are undeniable. It is never too late to practice; an appropriate diet during breastfeeding favors the child's growth and improves her cognitive development.

Now you have all the keys to start eating properly. At Veritas, we hope that with this post, we have helped you to understand the enormous benefits that a balanced diet has on your health and, above all, that we have inspired you to put it into practice.

CHAPTER 1

Low GI Diets And Its Importance

The glycemic index indicates the level of sugar that food provides, a fundamental measure for diabetics. However, everyone needs to consider this factor since a hypoglycemic diet can prevent or control type 1 and 2 diabetes, among many other benefits that we will learn about in the development of this chapter.

The glycemic index (GI) is a measure used to quantify the carbohydrates in food. It does not do it for its calories, but for its ability to increase our sugar levels.

To quantify the GI, how much glucose rises is compared to that provided by white bread, whose GI reference is 100.

Therefore, the GI is an important element in the control of diabetes. Is considered:

- A low GI when it is equal to or less than 55.
- The middle is between 56 and 69.
- High GI above 70.

Foods that have a GI greater than 70 and that must be kept under control are, of course, sugar or honey. There are also others not so obvious.

White rice, mashed potatoes, and white bread. And processed foods, in general, are best taken in moderation.
On the other hand, whole-grain rice and bread, and legumes (lentils, peas, chickpeas) are good ingredients in this ideal diet.

The diet also depends on the metabolism of each person to assimilate carbohydrates.

The diet must be different for each person since the diner matters and considers the menu, depending on your metabolism and the ability of your body to assimilate carbohydrates.

Eating on a low-carb diet doesn't have to be complicated. The nutritionist can give you a lot of useful advice. Here are some examples.

- Instead of potatoes, the sweet potato, which has a low GI, is better.
- Instead of the usual loaf, you can choose spelled or rye bread, which is very popular and easily available today.
- Fruits like apples and oranges have a lower GI than others.

As a rule, the more fiber an ingredient has, the slower its glucose production.

In no case should carbohydrates be eliminated? They are necessary, and too strict diets that seek to eliminate them are not healthy.

The low glycemic index diet is ideal for those who want to lose weight without calculating calories, without going hungry, and without getting depressed! But, above all, without recovering the lost kilos as soon as the diet ends.

The low glycemic index diet aims to carry out an intelligent diet that satisfies us but limits those foods that will accumulate as fat in the body.

The best thing about this diet? Many of our favorite foods, like cheese and chocolate, are allowed. Benefits: do not give up anything; lose weight in a lasting way.

To understand the low glycemic index diet, you must first banish a series of myths: no, there are no "bad sugars" (those in sweets, drinks...) and "good sugars" (those in bread, pasta, rice, cereals...). And it is not true that the former is systematically fattening, nor is the latter good for health. What matters, in this case, is the glycemic index (GI) of food, which is the rate at which the body assimilates it.

Glucose (sugar) has the highest glycemic index: 100. The closer a food's glycemic index is to 100, the more likely the body is to convert it to fat. On the contrary, the closer your index is to 0, the more your body will burn it, favoring weight loss. Discovering the GI of the main foods that contain sugar will help you understand the requirements that can be consumed during the diet and the requirements that can not.

If you want the low glycemic index diet to be effective, it is important to follow these rules:

- Give priority to carbohydrates with a low GI: you do not have to eliminate all foods containing sugars or starch, but you should give preference to those with a low glycemic index. Fruits and vegetables should be the carbohydrates with the most presence in your diet. In the case, for example, of pasta, you shouldn't cook it too much since it increases the GI. Also, opt for lentils and other legumes; they will nourish you and, at the same time, help you lose weight!

- Include protein in your meals: it is recommended that you include protein in the different meals of the day, be it breakfast, lunch, or dinner. You can eat eggs, meat, fish, or even cheese. Choose what you like best and vary. As for snacks during the day, around 11 a.m. and 5 p.m., it is recommended to opt for dried fruit (walnuts, hazelnuts, almonds…).

- Substitute animal fats for vegetable fats: these are better for health. To cook, it is always best to use extra virgin olive oil. And between the fat of meat or fish, it is preferable that of fish.

- Limit processed foods: the glycemic index of this type of food goes up a lot. We refer to those with added sugars, refined flours, and other not recommended compounds.

- Get moving: Regular physical activity will allow you to burn fat at exertion. It will also help increase your basal metabolism, which translates into less fat accumulation in the long term. Therefore, combine the diet with regular exercise (at least 30 minutes a day).

To get blood sugar to rise more gradually and thus avoid hyperglycemia (high blood sugar levels) when consuming foods rich in carbohydrates, Belén Siscar explains that we apply some of her advice already mentioned above to reduce the glycemic load of the food we eat:

Eat whole grains.
It is important to consume all the cereals in their integral format (rice, pasta, bread…), since when grinding the grain, the three parts are preserved: germ, endosperm, and bran, the latter being the "shell" of the cereal, which is very rich in fiber which causes the GI to be lower since digestion is slower, while after the refinement process practically only one part remains: the endosperm, very rich in starch.

Generate resistant starch.
A very effective and easy trick to reduce the GI is to generate resistant starch, which is also super beneficial for our intestinal microbiota. To generate it, we only have to cook carbohydrates-rich food (sweet potato, potato, rice…) and quickly cool it in the fridge (4-5°C). During this time, the starch will undergo a retrogradation process and become resistant to oxidation. After 12-24 hours, we can drink it, and it doesn't have to be cold; we can reheat it without going over the temperature because we can reverse the process.

Complete dishes.
It is important to cook complete dishes because, in addition to being nutritionally healthier, it will also help reduce the GI. "If we add protein to a plate of macaroni, such as prawns, we add a vegetable such as broccoli and cherry tomatoes, and a good drizzle of olive oil, we are going to

slow down digestion and, therefore, the release of sugar in the blood," he says. Therefore, combining foods rich in carbohydrates with protein, vegetables, and healthy fats is interesting.

Cooking.

How food is cooked also influences how quickly our blood sugar will rise. For example, cooking pasta al dente or paella to the point without the rice "exploding," in addition to being much tastier, is also more beneficial, since that point of cooking reduces the glycemic index compared to overcooking, "so It is better if it is a little "hard" but without going over.

Underripe fruit.

The ripening point of the fruit is also key because the less ripe the fruit is, the less sugar it contains. Therefore, the lower the GI.

CHAPTER 2

Mediterranean Diet

The Mediterranean diet is based on consuming fresh and natural foods such as olive oil, fruits, vegetables, legumes, nuts, vinegar, cereals, fish, milk, and cheese, which is necessary to avoid industrialized products such as sausages, frozen and prefabricated food.
This diet is a type of diet that helps change lifestyle, and it is not always necessary to be low in calories to help lose weight since it naturally helps improve metabolism and promote weight control.

Main benefits
The Mediterranean diet is not just a diet to lose weight; it is more of a lifestyle present in the countries around the Mediterranean Sea. Its main health benefits are:

- Lower risk of developing cardiovascular diseases, cancer, diabetes, and degenerative diseases
- Protects the body from atherosclerosis and thrombosis
- Contains more nutrients than industrialized foods, providing a greater amount of vitamins and minerals
- It makes food more varied, excellent for children's palates, making it easier to eat vegetables and salads.

To lead the lifestyle of the Mediterranean diet, you should consume fruits and foods of plant origin, fresh, unprocessed, of the season, and preferably locally produced daily. It is preferable to buy them in small markets or greengrocers.
To follow the Mediterranean diet, you must alter your diet in the following way:

Avoid industrialized products.
The diet should be mostly plant-based products, such as brown rice, soybeans, and legumes. However, natural animal products, such as eggs and milk can also be consumed in moderation. In addition, foods that were bought ready-made, such as cakes, should be avoided, giving preference to homemade versions.
Removing industrialized products will help reduce the production of toxins in the body, reduce inflammation, and combat fluid retention, naturally helping to reduce swelling.

Eat Fish.

Fish should be consumed at least three times a week. They are sources of protein and good fats such as omega-3, which acts as an anti-inflammatory, helping to relieve joint pain, improve blood circulation, increase good cholesterol, and decrease the risk of heart disease.

Olive Oil And Good Fats.

Olive oil and vegetable oils such as canola and flaxseed oil are rich in heart-healthy fats, helping control cholesterol and prevent cardiovascular disease. Olive oil should be added to ready meals to obtain the benefits, consuming two tablespoons per day.

Other sources of good fats are olives and nuts such as peanuts, walnuts, almonds, and hazelnuts, which should be consumed 1 to 2 servings per day.

Whole Foods.

The Mediterranean diet is rich in whole foods, including cereals such as oats, rye, and barley; Integral rice; wheat pasta; and wholemeal bread, which are foods rich in fiber, vitamins, and minerals that improve the functioning of the body, combat constipation and reduce the absorption of sugars and fats in the intestine.

In addition to this, it is also rich in high-protein grains like beans, soybeans, and chickpeas, which also help build muscle and improve metabolism.

Fruits And Vegetables.

Increasing the consumption of fruits and vegetables is an important point in this diet. They provide fibers, vitamins, and minerals for the body, causing a greater feeling of satiety and favoring weight loss.

Skimmed Milk And Derivatives.

To improve your diet and reduce your fat intake, you should prefer skim milk, natural yogurt, and white cheeses such as ricotta and cottage, or choose the low-fat versions of the products, always being careful to read the nutritional labeling.

Wine.

Drinking 30 cc of wine daily has been shown to help heart health due to its high polyphenols such as resveratrol, a substance rich in antioxidants, which helps take care of blood vessels. Alcohol in excess should be drunk in moderation; it negatively affects health.

CHAPTER 3

Glycemic Index Of Main Foods

The glycemic index (GI) is how food containing carbohydrates increases blood glucose, the amount of sugar in the blood once it is absorbed at the intestinal level.

For this reason, knowing the GI of certain foods is important to help control hunger, anxiety, increase the feeling of satiety, regulate blood glucose, help to control prediabetes and diabetes, and facilitate weight loss. Or help maintain it.

It is also important for athletes since it provides information on foods that help obtain energy or recover energy reserves, especially in high-impact sports.

Foods with a GI of less than 55 have a low glycemic index and are generally the healthiest; those between 56 and 69 have a moderate glycemic index, and foods with values above 70 have a high glycemic index and should normally be avoided in the diet or consumed in moderation.

The value of the glycemic index of foods is not calculated based on a portion. It compares the number of carbohydrates that food contains concerning glucose, whose GI is 100.

The table below includes the low, medium, and high GI carbohydrate foods most consumed by the general population:

Carbohydrate Rich Foods

Low GI ≤ 55	Medium GI 56-69	High GI ≥ 70
All-Bran: 30	Brown Rice: 68	White Rice: 73
Oatmeal: 54	Couscous: 65	Isotonic drinks such as Gatorade: 78
Milk chocolate: 43	Cassava flour: 61	Rice crackers: 87

Integral spaghetti: 49	Arepa (Corn flour): 60	corn cereal: 81
Rice noodles: 53	Popcorn: 65	White wheat bread: 75
Whole grain bread: 53	Soft drinks: 59	Tapioca: 70
Corn tortilla: 50	Muesli: 57	Cornstarch: 85
Barley: 30	Bread with grains: 53	Tacos: 70
Fructose: 15	Homemade pancakes: 66	Glucose: 103

Vegetables And Legumes (General Classification)

Low GI ≤ 55	Medium GI 56-69	High GI ≥ 70
Beans: 24	Steamed yams: 51	Mashed potatoes: 87
Lentils: 32	Cooked pumpkin: 64	Potato: 78
Cooked carrot: 39	Green banana: 55	-
Vegetable soup: 48	Turnips: 62	-
Cooked sweet corn: 52	Cassava: 55	-
Cooked soybeans: 20	Peas: 54	-
Grated raw carrot: 35	French fries: 63	-
Sweet potato with skin and cooked: 44	Beetroot: 64	-
Carob: 40	Sweet potatoes without skin: 61	-

The glycemic index can vary according to the type of fruit. In this way, the glycemic index of the main fruits consumed daily is indicated in the following table:

Fruits (General Classification)

Low GI ≤ 55	Medium GI 56-69	High GI ≥ 70
Apple: 36	Kiwi: 58	Watermelon: 76
Strawberries: 40	Papaya: 56	-
Orange: 43	Peach in syrup: 58	-
Unsweetened apple juice: 44	Pineapple: 59	-
Orange Juice: 50	Grapes: 59	-
Banana: 51	Black cherries: 63	-
Mango: 51	Melon: 65	-
Apricot: 34	Dates: 62	-
Peach: 28	Raisins: 64	-
Pear: 33	Blueberries: 53	-
-	Plums: 53	-

Oilseeds

Oilseeds, such as nuts and seeds, all have a low glycemic index; however, they must be consumed in moderation as they provide many calories.

It is important to remember that meals should be prepared with foods with a low or medium glycemic index. It reduces fat accumulation in the body, increases the feeling of satiety, and reduces hunger.

As for how much of the food should be ingested, this will depend on the calories that the individual needs to consume during the day; for this reason, it is important to go to a nutritionist to carry out a personalized nutritional evaluation and indicate which portions to ingest.

Glycemic Index Of Foods And Whole Meals
The glycemic index of whole meals is different from the glycemic index of single foods because, during the digestion of a meal, the foods mix and cause different effects on blood glucose. So if a meal is rich in carbohydrate foods such as bread, chips, soft drinks, and ice cream, it will have a greater ability to increase blood sugar, which has adverse health effects such as weight gain, cholesterol, and triglycerides.

On the other hand, a balanced and varied meal containing rice, beans, raw salad, meat, and olive oil will have a low glycemic index and keep blood sugar stable, bringing health benefits.
A good suggestion to balance meals is to include whole foods, fruits, vegetables, nuts such as peanuts and cashews, and protein sources such as milk, yogurt, eggs, and meats.

CHAPTER 4

Meal Plan

When we talk about a food plan, we refer to that guide that helps us control what we eat based on a healthy and balanced diet made from the body's basic needs.
Therefore, the food plan is carried out in a personalized way, according to the needs of each patient.

However, it also considers the person's lifestyle and eating habits in the same way.

What Is The Difference Between An Eating Plan And A Diet?

It should be noted that the main difference between a food plan and a diet is that the former is carried out in a personalized way since the tastes and conditions of the patient are considered individually.
While the diet is based on eliminating certain foods and their dosage for weight loss or maintenance.

How To Make A Food Plan?

As we mentioned before, the food plan is a personalized guide to lead a healthy life based on our diet.

This plan is developed taking into account:

- Age.
- Sex.
- Physical condition.
- Daily energy expenditure.
- Intolerances and allergies.
- Existing illness or disease.

The above is done to develop a food plan tailored to our patient, benefiting his body, mind, and health, noting the benefits and effects of a balanced diet.
If you have begun to be interested in improving your diet and don't know how to start, the advice we give you today on developing a healthy eating plan will be of great help. What should I do, and when should I eat it? What foods can I mix? How many times can I eat each food?...

First Step: Buy Healthy Food

The first step you must follow in a healthy eating plan is that the food part of your diet is healthy. In this way, it will be much easier for you to prepare a healthy weekly menu for the whole family, and you will avoid the temptation to eat unhealthy foods.

If you are wondering what kind of healthy foods you should include in your diet, here is a list of the different food groups that you should take into account when making your weekly purchase:

Vegetables. Surely we will not surprise you if we tell you that vegetables should be part of a balanced diet. They are very rich in vitamins, minerals, and fiber. Please make sure they are at least in your main meals. No vegetable or vegetable is better or worse than another. Each one will provide specific nutrients, so variety is the key. Make sure your dishes are full of color, and you can take advantage of all its benefits.

Fruit. Another classic that cannot be missing from a healthy and balanced diet is fruit. Try to consume 2 or 3 pieces of fruit a day. Like vegetables, fruits will also provide extra vitamins, fiber, and minerals to your diet. You can consume them between meals, as a dessert or as part of the main dish such as a salad. There are no rules or schedules for mixing and consuming the fruit!

Cereals and derivatives. Cereals and their derivatives are a source of carbohydrates for the diet, whose main function is to provide energy. You must choose the whole grain versions over the refined ones and avoid processed products such as cookies, pastries, or sugary cereals.
Healthy fats have been dismissed as "unhealthy" for a long time. However, healthy fats, unsaturated fats, should be part of a healthy diet. Some foods with healthy fats that should be part of your diet are nuts, seeds, olive oil, or avocado. On the contrary, try to limit the consumption of saturated fats present in fatty sausages, industrial pastries, salty snacks, etc.

Legumes and tubers. Legumes are often forgotten in our diet, but they are an excellent option for vegetable proteins. If you do not have time to cook them, you can buy the boats of cooked vegetables. In 5 minutes, you can have a delicious and nutritious salad. Tubers such as sweet potatoes or potatoes are also a good option to achieve different flavors and textures in the kitchen.

Dairy and vegetable equivalents. Dairy is a good source of calcium and quality protein to be part of a balanced and healthy diet. Plant-based equivalents like plant-based drinks or calcium-enriched plant-based yogurts are also a good option if you can't or choose not to eat dairy. It is important not to include dairy desserts such as custard, flan, ice cream... which are foods that are very rich in added sugar.

Meat, fish, seafood, and eggs. These food groups will provide you with good quality protein in your diet. Try to make them part of your main meals and avoid processed products of less nutritional quality, such as nuggets, fish sticks, frankfurter-type sausages, etc., unless homemade. Never forget that a healthy diet begins with the purchase of healthy foods.

Are Your Dishes Balanced?

Once we have made sure that the food at home is healthy, we will ensure that the dishes that make up your main meals are also healthy. To do this, we suggest you follow the plate method. It is about dividing your plate into three parts:

One-half of the plate is made up of vegetables. Vegetables will provide fiber, vitamins, and minerals to your recipes. The more variety of vegetables and vegetables you incorporate, the more variety of nutrients you can obtain.

A quarter of the plate consists of quality protein foods: lean meats, white fish, oily fish, eggs, legumes and tempeh, tofu, seitan.
A quarter of the plate consists of foods rich in carbohydrates: whole grains and derivatives, tubers, and legumes. Think that carbohydrates are our main source of energy, do not forget to incorporate them into your main meals.
Here are some ideas for dishes that follow the healthy plate method and that you can incorporate into your diet:

Planning A Healthy Weekly Menu

Now that you have mastered your plate let's go for the week. Weekly menu planning is complex, but we encourage you to start working on it. To do so, you can consult one of our publications on healthy weekly menus. You can also get help from other websites like the Seguros Catalana Occidente blog on nutrition.

To prepare a weekly plan, we must always keep in mind the idea of the dish. Always try to have a part of vegetables and vegetables, one of the protein foods and another of foods rich in carbohydrates. In order not to displace any food group, try to distribute the protein food group following the weekly consumption frequencies that we propose below:

- White meat: 3 times a week
- Red meat: maximum one time per week
- Whitefish: 3 times a week
- Bluefish: 1 – 2 times a week
- Legumes: minimum 2 – 3 times a week
- Seafood: 1 – 2 times per week
- Eggs: 2 – 3 times a week

Try to make the main cooking of your recipes healthy and moderate the fried and battered ones. Prioritize healthy cooking such as grilling, baking, steaming, boiling, sautéing, or healthy stews.

5 Weeks Meal Plan

You can find the meal plan recipes below in their respective section of the day.

WEEK 1

Day	Breakfast	Lunch	Dinner	Snack
Monday	Toast With Roasted Tomatoes And Crushed Avocado	Caesar Salad With Romaine Lettuce And Grilled Chicken	Margherita Pizza	White Bean Dip
Tuesday	German Pancakes	Grilled Chicken With Fresh Spinach and Tomato Confit	Pumpkin Gazpacho	Apple Crisp
Wednesday	Spanish Toast	Zucchini And Aubergines Stuffed With Tomato And Cheese	Tasty Beef and Broccoli	Cashew and Peanut Rice Pudding
Thursday	Mallorcan Empanadas	Chicken With Spinach And Lemon Cream	Pumpkin And Clove Cream With Kale Sprouts	Chocolate-Coated Dates
Friday	Muhammara	Grilled Chicken With Chanterelles and Pumpkin	Classic Pasta Amatriciana	Pumpkin Yogurt Parfait
Saturday	Tahini	Herbed Up Feisty Baby Potatoes	Baked Sea Bass With Oyster Mushrooms And Pickled Lemon	Roasted Peach and Orange Crostini
Sunday	Avocado Caprese Toast	Turkey Lasagna	Pork Potato	Cherry-Peach Compote with Greek Yogurt

WEEK 2

Day	Breakfast	Lunch	Dinner	Snack
Monday	Herbed Parmesan Walnuts	Cuttlefish Tagine With Lemon	Pork Chops and Tomato Sauce	Carrot Chips
Tuesday	Avocado and Blueberry Medley	Shrimp in White Wine	Hake With Tomatoes Marinated In Soy	Veggie Sushi
Wednesday	Cool Red Pepper and Olive Omelette	Cuttlefish Casserole With Mushrooms	Beef Corn Chili	Crispy BBQ Roasted Chickpeas
Thursday	Hearty Pumpkin Oats	Chicken With Spinach And Lemon Cream	Pumpkin Cream With Smoked Herring Roe And Black Garlic	Vegan Brownie Bites
Friday	Cheesy Zucchini Omelette	Cuttlefish Noodles With Shiitake And Parmesan	Fettuccine Pomodoro	Triple-Berry Smoothie Bowl
Saturday	Strawberry and Rhubarb Smoothie	Spanish paella	Baked Sea Bass With Potatoes And Spring Garlic	Baked Popcorn Chicken
Sunday	Barley Porridge	Chicken Skewers With Satay Sauce	Rosemary Beef Chuck Roast	Roasted Pepper And Eggplant

WEEK 3

Day	Breakfast	Lunch	Dinner	Snack
Monday	Refreshing Mango and Pear Smoothie	Italian Chicken	Grilled Sea Bream With Clams	Fava Bean Guacamole With Root Chips
Tuesday	Breakfast Quinoa	Bruschetta With Balsamic Dressing, Olives, And Pepper	Soy Sauce Beef Roast	Rainbow Heirloom Tomato Bruschetta
Wednesday	Almond Risotto	Cuttlefish Skewers With Romesco Sauce	Low-Temperature Teriyaki Cod	Roasted Veggie Chips
Thursday	Garlic Eggs	Chicken Stuffed With Kale And Toum Sauce	Pumpkin And Turnip Cream	Beet Hummus
Friday	Almond Risotto	Mediterranean Cheese	Pasta Con Pomodoro E Basilico	Healthy Lemon Bars
Saturday	Fresh Cheese with Tomato	Cuttlefish With Pickled Courgette	Salmon With Broccoli And Almond Cream	Falafel Smash
Sunday	Banana Nut Muffins	Mediterranean Kale Dish	Beef Corn Chili	All-Green Crudités Basket

WEEK 4

Day	Breakfast	Lunch	Dinner	Snack
Monday	Oatmeal Smoothie	Hot Spinach And Artichoke Cups	Tasty Beef and Broccoli	Blueberry Coconut Energy Bites
Tuesday	Mediterranean Breakfast With Pita Bread	Chicken Breast With Fennel Salad	Roasted Pumpkin Cream with Sage	Grab-and-Go Snack Jars
Wednesday	Easy Muesli	Asparagus Skewer And Cuttlefish Carpaccio With Parmesan	Balsamic Beef Dish	Smoked Salmon and Avocado Summer Rolls
Thursday	Spinach And Feta Breakfast Roll	Chicken Breast With Boletus And Spinach	Pumpkin Cream With Mi Cuit Foie And Black Truffle	Baked Beet Chips
Friday	Avocado Caprese Toast	Turkey Verde with Brown Rice	Mushroom Risotto	Fruicuterie Board
Saturday	Artichoke And Spinach Frittata	Chicken With Lemon And Hot Spices	Bean Salad With Avocado, Tomato And Sweet And Sour Radishes	Grilled Flatbread with Burrata Cheese
Sunday	Bean Salad With Avocado And Quinoa	Cuttlefish With Ginger And Coconut Milk	Salmon With Sesame And Orange	White Bean Dip

WEEK 5

Day	Breakfast	Lunch	Dinner	Snack
Monday	Egg And Mushrooms On Toast	Cuttlefish Tagine With Lemon	Pork Chops and Tomato Sauce	Apple Crisp
Tuesday	Broccoli & Eggs	Shrimp Bruschetta With Orzo Pasta	Hake With Tomatoes Marinated In Soy	Tomato, Avocado, Egg And Sweet And Sour Cucumber Sandwich
Wednesday	Coconut Risotto	Salad With Chickpeas, Bulgur, And Orange	Soy Sauce Beef Roast	White Bean And Bacon Dip
Thursday	Power Packed Oatmeal	Aubergine Flatbread With Roasted Garlic And Sepionets	Pumpkin Cream With Roasted Chickpeas And Avocado	Avocado, Mozzarella, And Roasted Pepper Pate Sandwich
Friday	Labneh With Garlic And Mint	Grilled Chicken With Bimi, Soy Sauce And Kimchi	Pasta Carbonara	Ham And Brie Cheese Piadina
Saturday	Tangerine, Cocoa And Evoo Muffins	Sautéed Chickpeas With Cuttlefish	Salmon With Broccoli And Almond Cream	Crispy And Spicy Chickpeas
Sunday	Avocado Caprese Toast	Turkey Meatloaf	Grilled Sea Bream With Clams	Carrot Chips

CHAPTER 5

Breakfast

What Should A Balanced And Healthy Mediterranean Breakfast Contain?

The **Mediterranean breakfast usually** includes coffee, infusions, milk with cocoa, natural orange juice, toast with olive oil and tomato, sausages, fruit, and yogurt. These are some of the essentials of Mediterranean food that cannot be missing from a balanced Mediterranean breakfast.

1. **Healthy fats**: The queen of healthy fats is virgin olive oil, the star of Mediterranean cuisine. Essential in our toasts in the morning.
2. **Carbohydrates:** we will find them in bread and cereals. Suppose they are integral, better.
3. Calcium: milk, yogurts, or cheese. We can add cheese to the toast or prepare yogurt with honey and cereal.
4. **Proteins of high biological value**: if we add a slice of quality Serrano ham to our toast with oil and tomato, we will have proteins, which will be key to preventing us from feeling hungry again shortly after breakfast.
5. **Vitamins and fiber:** fruits will provide us with the vitamins we need: from the tomato on toast to a kiwi, melon, pineapple... Be careful with orange juice. Although it is healthy and provides us with vitamin C, we lose a good part of the fiber, which remains in the skin and pulp when squeezing the orange.
6. **Caffeine:** coffee and tea: they provide us with doses of caffeine that, in the right measure, are very beneficial for the body, especially at the beginning of the day.

Recipes

Mediterranean Pita With Chicken, Bell Pepper Andra, mean Roasted Garlic

Ingredients for two portions

Pepper sauce

- 2 cups red bell peppers
- 1 cup eggplant, diced
- 1 Roma tomato, quartered
- six garlic cloves, whole (unpeeled)
- two tablespoons olive oil
- $\frac{1}{3}$ cup fresh parsley, chopped
- $\frac{1}{2}$ lemon, just the juice
- sea salt, to taste
- pepper, to taste

Chicken

- 9 oz (250g) lean chicken drumsticks (unprocessed)
- one teaspoon olive oil

To serve

- two whole-grain Arabic pieces of bread
- three tablespoons Greek yogurt
- 2 cups of mixed vegetables
- fresh coriander

STEPS

Set an oven to 400°F / 200°C.
Arrange bell pepper, eggplant and tomato, and whole garlic cloves on a baking sheet.
Drizzle with half the olive oil, salt, and pepper. Roast for 15-20
minutes until the pepper is blistered, slightly charred, and softened.
While the vegetables are roasting, it's time to prepare the chicken. Heat a skillet (or frying pan) over high heat. Toss the chicken in a little olive oil and seasoning. Place the chicken in the pan and brown for 3-4 minutes. Turn and repeat until browned and cooked through.
Remove the baking sheet with vegetables from the oven. Let cool for a few minutes before handling. Squeeze the garlic cloves out of the skin and transfer them to a clean cutting board with the remaining vegetables. Chop and puree together. You can add this mixture to a food processor while cooking a large batch.
Transfer to a bowl and add chopped parsley, lemon juice, and remaining olive oil. Mix, taste, and adjust the seasoning if necessary.
To assemble, heat the pita bread. Top with a portion of the roasted pepper sauce, salad, and grilled chicken. Drizzle on Greek yogurt and enjoy!
If meal prepping, place chicken, yogurt, salad, and roasted pepper sauce in meal prep containers. Wrap the pita separately and assemble just before eating.

Toast With Roasted Tomatoes And Crushed Avocado

Ingredients for two portions

- 10.5 ounces (300g) cherry tomatoes, on the vine (preferred)
- one tablespoon extra virgin olive oil
- sea salt, to taste
- pepper, to taste
- 1 avocado
- 2 eggs
- 2 slices whole wheat bread

STEPS

Set oven to 350°F / 180°C.
Toss tomato halves in olive oil and seasoning. Transfer to a baking sheet in an even layer and bake for 20-25 minutes, until soft and fragrant.
Meanwhile, bring water to a boil in a pot, gently add the eggs and cook for 6 minutes to get soft-cooked eggs. Remove and plunge into ice water to prevent further cooking. Then peel.
Toast whole wheat bread. Top with avocado, juicy roasted tomatoes, hard-boiled eggs, and a generous sprinkle of salt and pepper.
I recommend heating the tomatoes and toasting the bread before assembling to prepare the meal. Depending on how much time you have in the mornings, you can even boil the eggs ahead of time and store them in the fridge.

Roasted Almond Honey Bars

Ingredients for 8 bars

- ¾ cup of rolled oats
- ½ cup almonds, toasted
- ⅓ cup of raisins
- ½ teaspoon ground cinnamon
- ½ cup peanut butter, or your choice of nut or seed butter
- ¼ cup of organic raw honey

STEPS

Tip: First, toast the almonds. This brings out the nuts' oi transforms the flavor, so it's worth the extra minute.
Place the walnuts in a dry skillet over medium heat, stirring every few seconds until they smell toasty and brown.
Let cool, and then chop the almonds. Mix with the other dry ingredients (oats, raisins, cinnamon).
In a separate bowl, mix the peanut butter and honey. If it's hard to mix, put it in the microwave for 10 seconds to soften.
Add the dry ingredients to the honey and peanut butter mixture and stir until no dry oats remain.
Line a loaf tin with baking paper, about 8 x 2 inches (20 x 5 cm) in size. Or drizzle with olive oil. Transfer the mixture to the lined baking sheet. Press down with the back of a spoon to compact the mixture. Place in the fridge for an hour or overnight. Then remove, cut into portions and wrap.

Note: I like to store these bars in the freezer to avoid temptation so that I can make a really big batch. Still, there will be fine in a sealed container at room temperature for 5-6 days.

Chickpea And Spinach Stew
Main ingredients

- one tablespoon olive oil
- 5.3 ounces (150g) onion, diced
- two cloves garlic, finely chopped
- ½ tablespoon smoked paprika
- ½ teaspoon ground cumin
- two tablespoons tomato paste
- 3 ½ cups vegetable stock / 830 ml
- 10.5 ounces (300g) chickpeas, canned
- 7 ounces (200g) red potatoes, diced
- ¼ lemon, (use a peeler to remove two large pieces of skin)
- one bay leaf (optional)
- 2 cups spinach, raw

Decorate

- fresh parsley
- ½ lemon, just the juice
- two teaspoons extra virgin olive oil
- one tablespoon chopped almonds

STEPS

Place a large, deep pot over medium heat. Add olive oil, onion, and garlic. Season with salt. This is the key to an amazing Spanish stew. Wait about 10 minutes for the onion and garlic to turn translucent slowly and softly; if they start to color, reduce the heat. Add smoked paprika and cumin. Stir. Next, add the tomato paste and cook, stirring for 2 minutes.

Add the vegetable broth, chickpeas, potato, bay leaf, and lemon zest. Bring to a simmer and cook for 20 minutes until the potato is cooked through and the flavors have developed.

Finally, add the spinach. Stir to wilt. Then remove from heat. Find and remove any large pieces of lemon zest or skin.
Serve and garnish with lemon juice, olive oil, flaked almonds, and fresh parsley.

German Pancakes Recipe

Ingredients

- 1 ¼ Cup - Milk
- 4 Eggs
- 1 Cup - Flour
- ¼ Teaspoon Salt
- Butter
- Fillings of Choice: Cinnamon and Sugar; Jams; Jellies, Fruit, etc.
- Powdered Sugar (Optional)
- Syrup (optional).

STEPS

Crack open the eggs into a bowl.
Add Milk to eggs; beat well.
Mix Flour and Salt in a separate bowl.
Stir flour and salt mixture into the milk and eggs gradually, until smooth.
The batter will be thin.
Heat a heavy 8-inch to 10-inch skillet and grease lightly with butter or oil.
Pour only enough batter to make a very thin pancake. Tip the skillet from side to side and around to help spread the pancake batter as needed.

Cook on one side (without flipping) until the pancake begins to blister or bubble. Flip the pancake and cook the other side until a light golden color. Do not overcook. You do not want them to get hard or crispy. NOTE: Pancakes cook very quickly; pay attention. Remove from the skillet and place it aboard. Once you have several pancakes stacked on the board, you can begin filling one at a time. Brush one side only with butter.
Add about 1 to 2 Tablespoons (s) of your desired filling: Cinnamon and Sugar; Jam; Jelly; Fruit; etc. to the buttered side.
Roll pancake from one edge across to the other side.
Place rolled pancake (or two) on a plate and dust with Powdered Sugar.

Lebanese Cheese Fatayers

Ingredients for the mass:

- 1 ¼ cup organic whole wheat flour
- 5 ounces (150 g) organic white flour
- 150 ml (5.4 fl oz) warm water
- 2 teaspoons baker's yeast powder
- 1 teaspoon of sea salt

For the cheese filling:
- 8.8 ounces (250 g) feta cheese
- 1 teaspoon dried mint

STEPS

Mix the flour, salt, and yeast in a large bowl. Make a hole in the center and pour the olive oil and warm water. With a silicone spatula, mix the flour well with the liquid. Work the mixture well and continue kneading with your hands until you obtain a soft and hydrated dough that does not stick.

Cover the bowl with a cloth and place it in a warm place in the house for at least half an hour until the dough has doubled in volume. Remove the dough from the bowl and place it on a clean and previously floured worktop. Knead a little with your hands and, with the help of a rolling pin (lightly dusted with flour), gradually roll out the dough.
With the help of a small square cutter (approx. 7cm - 2.75 inches), make small portions of dough, and they will be ready to fill with the cheese filling.
For the cheese filling:
In a bowl, mix the feta cheese with the teaspoon of dry mint with the help of a fork.
For the final preparation:
Preheat the oven to 175 degrees C /350 degrees F.
To fill small portions of dough, add one teaspoon of the cheese filling to the center of the dough, making sure to keep the sides of the dough clean.
Fold the square portion of dough starting at each corner, joining the four sides of the dough, making sure to close and press the edges well so they do not open.
Bake in the middle of the oven for about 20 minutes at 350 degrees °F /175 degrees °C until the crust is golden brown.
Remove from the oven and enjoy hot or cold.

Vegan Pesto Manchego Empanada

Ingredients

For the dough (Multipurpose olive oil dough)
- 150 g / 1 ¼ cup organic whole wheat flour
- 150 g / 1 ¼ cup organic white flour

- 75 ml /2.7 fl oz extra virgin olive oil (EVOO)
- 150 ml / 5.4 fl oz warm water
- 2 teaspoons of powdered baker's yeast
- 1 teaspoon of sea salt

For the Manchego ratatouille
- 2 tablespoons of extra virgin olive oil (EVOO)
- 2 garlic cloves peeled and finely chopped
- 1 medium onion peeled and finely chopped
- one red bell pepper, seeded and diced
- one green bell pepper, seeded and diced
- 1 Zucchini, diced
- ½ teaspoon of pimentón de la vera (Spanish paprika)
- 6 medium tomatoes, peeled and diced (if tomatoes are not in season, you can use 1 pound 12 ounces / 800 g tomato passata)
- one teaspoon sea salt (or salt to taste)

STEPS

For the dough (multipurpose olive oil dough)

Mix the flour, salt, and yeast in a large bowl. Make a hole in the center and pour the olive oil and warm water. With a silicone spatula, mix the flour well with the liquid. Work the mixture well and continue kneading with your hands until you obtain a soft and hydrated dough that does not stick.
Cover the bowl with a cloth and place it in a warm place in the house for at least half an hour until the dough has doubled in volume. Remove the dough from the bowl and place it on a clean and previously floured worktop.

For the Pesto Manchego

Have all the vegetables well washed and prepared as indicated in the description of the ingredients.
In a pan with a lid, heat the olive oil (2 tablespoons), add the garlic and fry for 1 minute until lightly browned. Then add the onion, red and green peppers, and a pinch of salt and fry over medium heat for about 5 minutes until soft but not toasty. Add the zucchini and stir for another minute.
Reduce heat to low temperature. Add the ½ teaspoon of Pimentón de la Vera (Spanish Paprika), the tomatoes, and a teaspoon of salt and stir. Cook, covered with a lid, over medium-low heat for about 15 minutes, stirring occasionally. Remove from heat and let cool.

For the final preparation

Preheat the oven to 175 degrees °C /350 degrees °F.
Knead a little with your hands, cut the dough into two portions and gradually roll out the dough on a clean surface with the help of a rolling pin (lightly dusted with flour). Line a medium-sized baking dish with non-stick baking paper. Place one of the portions on the baking paper and continue spreading it with your hands until you reach all the corners of the baking dish.
Add 400g /14 ounces of ratatouille from La Mancha and spread it out, leaving about 6 cm (2.4 inches) on the edges.
Add the other portion of the dough on top and glue the edges; close them well, so they do not open. Shape the edges by pinching them with your fingers. Use a fork to poke a few holes in the lid to allow steam to escape.

Bake in the middle of the oven for about 30 minutes at 350 degrees °F /175 degrees °C until the empanada is golden brown.

You can have it as a main dish adding a salad. If you have a little dough left, you can cut it into pieces and use it to decorate the empanada.

Blackberry, Banana And Yogurt Popsicles

Ingredients
- 1 cup blackberries
- 1 ripe banana, peeled and cut into small pieces
- 125 g / 6 tablespoons organic plain yogurt or your favorite plant-based plain yogurt
- 100 ml / $\frac{1}{2}$ cup of water

STEPS

Wash the blackberries well with cold water and drain.
Beat the blackberries, banana, yogurt, and water well with a mixer until smooth.
Pour the mixture into the popsicle molds with sticks and freeze for 4 hours.
Grades.
The preparation time is only 10 minutes, there is no cooking time, but it must be frozen for 3-4 hours.
If you are vegan or lactose intolerant, you can substitute plain yogurt for your favorite plant-based plain yogurt.

EVOO and yogurt cake
Ingredients

- 4 organic eggs
- 100 g / $\frac{1}{2}$ cup demerara or panela sugar or any variety of unrefined sugar
- 75 ml /2.7 fl oz extra virgin olive oil (EVOO)
- 125 g /5 tablespoons of natural organic yogurt. If you are lactose intolerant, you can replace it with your favorite plain plant-based yogurt
- 100 g / $\frac{3}{4}$ cup organic wholemeal flour
- 70 g / $\frac{1}{2}$ cup organic flour
- A pinch of sea salt
- 1 tablespoon of baking powder

STEPS

Preheat the oven to 175 degrees °C / 350 degrees °F.
Line a baking pan with parchment paper.
In a large bowl, beat the eggs with a mixer. Add the sugar and continue mixing until dissolved. Next, add the extra virgin olive oil and natural yogurt.
Add the flours, yeast, and salt. Mix well until all ingredients are well combined.
Fill the pan with the mixture and bake in the middle of the oven for about 40 minutes at 350 degrees °F / 175 degrees °C until a toothpick or thin skewer inserted into the middle of the cake comes out clean.
Remove from the oven and let cool on a rack.

Spanish Toast

Ingredients

- 6 thick slices of bread (preferably day-old bread)
- 3 tablespoons of brown sugar

- 2 cups skimmed milk (if you are lactose intolerant, you can substitute your preferred non-fat milk)
- 2 cinnamon sticks
- The skin of an organic lemon (avoid the bitter white membrane under the skin of the lemon)
- 2 Eggs

For Topping
- 2 tablespoons of brown sugar
- 1 tablespoon of cinnamon powder

STEPS

In a saucepan, add the milk, then three tablespoons of brown sugar, the two cinnamon sticks, and the skin of an organic lemon. Before it reaches the boiling point, stop the fire. Let the milk infuse until lukewarm. (If you wish, you can leave it to infuse for about an hour)

Beat the eggs on a deep plate.

In another deep dish, add the infused milk and submerge each slice of bread in the milk. Please do not leave it too long in the milk. Otherwise, the bread risks breaking. Drain a little of the milk from the bread and add it to the plate of beaten eggs. Repeat the process with each slice of bread.

Preheat the oven to 175 degrees °C / 350 degrees °F. Add the torrijas to a deep oven dish. Bake in the middle of the oven for 10 minutes at 175 degrees °C /350 degrees °F. After those 10 minutes, turn each French toast and bake for ten more minutes until the French toast is golden.

Once golden, remove them from the oven and let them stay warm.

Add two tablespoons of brown sugar and a tablespoon of cinnamon powder on a deep plate. Mix well and sprinkle over the baked French toast.

Tangerine, Cocoa And Evoo Muffins

Ingredients

- 4 organic eggs
- $1/2$ cup (100 g) raw cane sugar
- 75 ml (2.7 fl oz) extra virgin olive oil (EVOO)
- 75 ml (2.7 fl oz) freshly squeezed mandarin orange juice
- 100 g ($3/4$ cup) organic flour
- 70 g ($1/2$ cup) organic wholemeal flour
- 3 tablespoons of raw cocoa 100%
- A pinch of sea salt
- 2 teaspoons of chemical yeast powder
- The zest of an organic tangerine (avoid the bitter white membrane under the tangerine rind)

STEPS

Preheat the oven to 175 degrees °C / 350 degrees °F.

In a muffin tray, place the muffin papers, or if you prefer not to use papers, lightly grease the muffin tray with olive oil and set it aside.

In a large bowl, beat the eggs with a mixer. Add the sugar and continue mixing until dissolved. Next, add the olive oil, the freshly squeezed mandarin juice, and the mandarin zest.

Next, add the flours, the yeast, the raw cocoa, and a pinch of salt and mix everything well until all the ingredients are well combined.

Fill the molds up to $3/4$ of their capacity.

Place the muffin pan in the middle of the oven and bake at 350 degrees °F /175 degrees °C for about 18 minutes. Remove from the oven and let cool.

Labneh With Garlic And Mint

Ingredients

- 500g (2 cups) organic Labneh (or thick organic plain yogurt like Greek yogurt)
- 3 garlic cloves, peeled and minced
- 1 ½ teaspoon dried mint
- 1 tablespoon of extra virgin olive oil (EVOO)
- A pinch of salt (or salt to taste)

STEPS

Mix the peeled and crushed garlic cloves, the pinch of salt, and the dry mint in a mortar until you get a paste.
Add the mixture to the labneh, mix well and sprinkle with a little EVOO.

Vegan Chickpea And Chocolate Cookies

Ingredients

- 250 g (1 ½ cups) organic chickpeas, cooked, drained, and rinsed
- 50g (½ cup) organic whole grain oat flakes (gluten-free)
- 75g (1/3 cup) unrefined brown sugar (demerara sugar, muscovado sugar, or coconut sugar)
- 3 tablespoons of organic pure cocoa powder
- 3 tablespoons of extra virgin olive oil (EVOO)
- 1 teaspoon of orange blossom water
- ½ teaspoon baking powder
- A pinch of sea salt

STEPS

Preheat the oven to 175 degrees °C / 350 degrees °F.
Add all ingredients to a food processor and blend until smooth and even. With your hands, create a ball with the obtained dough. Place the dough ball on parchment paper and cover it with another. Roll out the dough with the help of a rolling pin until it is the thickness of a €1 coin (approximately 0.25 cm). Cut out as many cookies as possible using a cookie-cutter but keep them slightly apart. Knead the rest of the cuts into a new ball and roll it out again using the same method with the baking paper.
Once all the cookies are cut, move the baking paper containing the cookies to the baking tray. I like to work directly on the parchment paper as it avoids the risk of breaking the cookies when I move them to the baking sheet.
Bake the cookies for about 20 minutes at 175 degrees °C /350 degrees °F. Remove from the oven and place on a cooling rack to cool completely before serving.

Muhammara

Ingredients

- 100g (1 cup) wholemeal breadcrumbs (you can grate some wholemeal bread leftover from the day before)
- 125g (1 cup) walnuts, peeled and chopped
- 2 large fresh red bell peppers
- 2 tablespoons of pine nuts
- 3 tablespoons pomegranate molasses

- 4 tablespoons of extra virgin olive oil (EVOO)
- 1 teaspoon cumin powder
- A pinch of freshly ground black pepper
- A pinch of salt (or salt to taste)
- ¼ cup (60 ml) water
- A pinch of spicy Vera paprika

STEPS

Have all the ingredients prepared as indicated in the description of the ingredients.
Preheat the oven to 200 degrees °C /392 degrees °F.
Wash the red peppers well, cut them in half, and remove the stems and seeds.
Lightly grease a baking dish with EVOO, place the cut red peppers, and skin side up. Roast for 15 minutes at 200°C / 392°F until the skin is lightly toasted. Remove the peppers from the oven, place them in a container, and cover them with plastic wrap. Once they are cool enough to handle, peel them and discard the skin.
With the help of a hand mixer or food processor, add the rest of the ingredients to the roasted red peppers and mix them all until you get a smooth paste. Serve in small bowls, sprinkle a little EVOO on top, and decorate with some nuts.

Mallorcan Empanadas

Ingredients

For the carrots dough:

- ¾ cup (175 ml) extra virgin olive oil (EVOO)
- ¾ cup (175 ml) lukewarm water
- 210g (1 ½ cup) organic wheat flour
- 210g (1 ½ cup) organic wholemeal flour

For the carrots filling:
- 1 tablespoon of extra virgin olive oil (EVOO)
- 1 small onion, peeled and finely chopped.
- 2 medium potatoes, peeled and finely diced
- 150g (1 cup) peas (fresh or frozen)
- 1 teaspoon sea salt (or salt to taste)
- 1 teaspoon of Vera paprika (optional)

STEPS

For the carrots dough:

Pour the warm water and the EVOO into a large container and add the flours. With a silicone spatula, mix the flour well with the liquid. Work the mixture well and continue kneading with your hands until you obtain a soft and hydrated dough that does not stick. Add a little extra flour if necessary.
Remove the dough from the bowl and place it on a clean surface dusted with flour. Knead a little with your hands and, with the help of a rolling pin (lightly dusted with flour), gradually roll out the dough. Once you have spread out the dough, with the help of a round cookie cutter (approx 15 cm - 6 inches in diameter), cut small round portions of dough and leave them ready to be filled.

For the carrots filling:

Have the vegetables well washed and prepared as indicated in the description of the ingredients.

In a container, add the peas, the potatoes, and the onions (all raw), the tablespoon of EVOO, salt to taste, and optionally the paprika. Mix everything well and reserve.

For the final preparation:

To fill small portions of dough, add one tablespoon of the filling to the center of the dough, making sure to keep the edges of the dough clean.

Fold the round portion of dough over the filling, adhere to the edges by supporting them with your fingers, making sure that they close well so that they do not open. Shape the edges by pinching with your fingers.

Preheat the oven to 175 degrees °C /350 degrees °F. Bake in the center of the oven for about 30 minutes at 350 degrees °F /175 degrees °C until the empanadas are golden brown.

Tahini

Ingredients

- 2 cups of vanilla yogurt
- 1 cup of boiling water
- 1 cup of crushed ice eight dates (chopped and pitted)
- $1/4$ cup of tahini
- 2 g of ground cinnamon (1 teaspoon)
- 1 g of Himalayan salt (1/5 teaspoon)

STEPS

Place the yogurt in an empty ice cube tray and freeze for 4 hours.

In a bowl, mix the dates and the boiling water, let them rest for 10 minutes, and then blend them until the mixture is smooth. Add frozen yogurt cubes, crushed ice, tahini, cinnamon, and Himalayan salt to a blender and date mixture.

Blend until smooth, serve in glasses and enjoy.

Artichoke And Spinach Frittata

Ingredients

- 10 eggs
- $1/2$ cup sour cream
- 1 tablespoon Dijon mustard
- 14 ounces (400 g) marinated artichoke hearts, drained, dried, and chopped
- 1 teaspoon kosher salt
- $1/4$ teaspoon black pepper
- 1 cup grated Parmesan cheese
- 5 ounces (140 g) spinach
- 2 cloves of minced garlic.

STEPS

You will start preparing this delicacy by preheating the oven to 200 °F (100 °C) with the rack in the middle. Place the eggs, sour cream, mustard, salt, pepper, and 1/2 cup Parmesan cheese in a large bowl or container and whisk to combine.

Heat oil in a nonstick skillet, which you can then take to the oven over medium heat and add the artichokes in a single layer. Cook, occasionally stirring until lightly browned. This can take you about 6 or 8 minutes. This will add the spinach and garlic to the pan until all the liquid evaporates. Spread everything out in an even layer and pour the egg mixture over the vegetables. Sprinkle with half a cup of Parmesan cheese and cook without stirring until the eggs are ready.

Balsamic Berries With Honey Yogurt

Ingredients

- 8 ounces (230 g) strawberries, halved
- 1 cup of blueberries
- 2/3 cup plain Greek yogurt
- 1 cup of raspberries
- 2 teaspoons of honey
- 1 tablespoon of balsamic vinegar.

STEPS

You will start this simple and delicious recipe by mixing the strawberries, blueberries, and raspberries with balsamic vinegar in a large bowl. Then let them rest for 10 minutes. Mix the yogurt and honey in a separate bowl and take your berry preparation to a serving plate; add a tablespoon of the previous mixture. And so enjoy a morning full of flavor.

Avocado Caprese Toast

Ingredients
- 2 slices of whole wheat bread
- 1 medium avocado cut in half and sliced
- 8 cherry tomatoes cut in half
- 2 bite-size mozzarella balls
- 4 fresh basil leaves
- 2 tablespoons balsamic vinegar

STEPS

This recipe will be as simple as toasting the bread and mashing the avocado in a small bowl. Spread the mashed avocado on the toast and cover it with cherry tomato slices, mozzarella cheese balls, and basil leaves. Finally, spread a little balsamic vinegar and start a morning full of energy just like that with this delicious Mediterranean breakfast.

Spinach And Feta Breakfast Roll

Ingredients
- 10 eggs
- ½ pound (90 g) of spinach
- 4 whole wheat tortillas
- ½ cup of cherry tomatoes
- 4 ounces (110 g) feta cheese
- extra virgin olive oil
- Salt and pepper to taste.

STEPS

You will start this recipe by putting a pan on the burner over medium heat, adding a splash of olive oil, and pouring in the eggs, occasionally stirring, until they are cooked. Season and reserve.
Put a tortilla on your work surface and add a quarter of each ingredient, including the eggs, spinach, tomato, and feta cheese. This is how you should wrap it to create a roll and repeat the process with the rest of the tortillas. You can eat it right there or store it in the refrigerator to warm it up the next morning.

Easy Muesli

Ingredients

- ½ cup of wheat bran
- ¼ cups of chopped walnuts
- ½ tablespoon kosher salt
- ¼ cup coarsely chopped dried apricots
- ½ teaspoon ground cinnamon
- 3 ½ cups of rolled oats
- ½ cup sliced almonds
- ¼ shelled pumpkin seeds
- ½ cup unsweetened coconut flakes
- ¼ cup of dried cherries.

STEPS

You will start this preparation by toasting the grains, nuts, and seeds in a tray on the lower rack. In another, you should put the oats, wheat bran, salt, and cinnamon on the top rack. Both trays should be in the oven for 10 or 12 minutes at 180 degrees.
Then, reserve the tray with nuts and add the coconut to the oatmeal tray to take it to the oven for five more minutes. Remove the last tray from the oven.
Once all the ingredients are cold, transfer them to a large bowl and add the nuts to integrate them into the mixture. You can store your muesli in an airtight container and enjoy it for a month.

Egg Toast With Lemon Yogurt

Ingredients

- 8 hard-boiled eggs
- 1 clove garlic
- 1 lemon
- 2 tablespoons finely chopped fresh dill
- ¾ teaspoon kosher salt
- two tablespoons finely chopped fresh chives
- ½ teaspoon freshly ground black pepper
- 2 cups plain Greek yogurt
- 4 slices of bread
- 2 tablespoons extra virgin olive oil
- 4 tablespoons of margarine without salt.

STEPS

Add the minced garlic clove, the grated lemon peel, and its juice in a bowl. Add the dill, basil, and fresh chives, the two cups of yogurt, two tablespoons of extra virgin olive oil, ¾ of kosher salt, and ½ teaspoon of black pepper. Thus, stir everything until the ingredients are combined.
Use the margarine and a hot skillet to brown the bread on both sides. Once you have the toasted bread, spread the yogurt mixture on the toast and add two eggs, which you will then crush with the wide part. Sprinkle a little salt and pepper to your liking to enjoy.

Mediterranean Breakfast With Pita Bread

Ingredients

- 4 boiled eggs
- 2 whole wheat pita bread cut in half

- ½ cup hummus
- 1 medium cucumber cut into thin slices
- 2 medium tomatoes
- 1 handful of fresh parsley leaves, coarsely chopped
- Hot sauce (optional)
- Salt and pepper to taste.

STEPS

Starting this preparation will be as simple as opening the bag created in your pita bread and filling it with two tablespoons of hummus, a slice of cucumber, a little tomato, and a sliced egg. Sprinkle your pita sandwich with a little parsley, salt, and pepper to taste. If you like breakfasts with a spicy touch, add hot sauce to your preparation and thus enjoy a perfect start.

Oatmeal Smoothie

Ingredients

- 1 cup (250 ml) of water
- 3 tbsp. raw oatmeal
- 1 small apple peeled and sliced
- 1 thin slice of ginger root

STEPS

Mix the ingredients in the blender.
Serve immediately.

Bean Salad With Avocado And Quinoa

Ingredients

- ½ cup of cooked beans
- Chicken soup
- A pinch of chives
- pepper to taste
- A pinch of salt
- 1 tbsp. Of olive oil
- ¼ avocado
- 1 tbsp lemon juice
- one sprig of coriander
- ½ cup of quinoa
- 1 tomato

STEPS

Combine the quinoa and chicken broth in a pot, bring to a boil, lower the heat, cover and cook for 15 minutes.
Transfer the quinoa to a bowl and let cool.
Add the beans, tomato, chives, lemon juice, avocado, and olive oil and stir.
Season with salt and pepper.
Decorate with the coriander.

Bread With Tomato, Oil, And Garlic

Ingredients

- one ripe tomato spread
- one slice of bread of splendid size (better if it is farmhouse bread or toasted rustic bread)
- Olive oil
- a bit of salt
- Garlic

STEPS

To be able to make this recipe, we will start by cutting the tomato in half without removing the skin
We take one of the halves, we face it with the crumb of the bread
We spread by pressing the content of the tomato strongly through the slice until it is completely red.

Mediterranean Salad

Ingredients

- 2 cups cucumber, peeled, seeded, diced
- 2 small red tomatoes, in squares
- 1 green bell pepper, diced
- 1/5 cup of red onion, in thin slices or half-moons
- 1/5 cup sliced black olives
- 1/5 cup feta cheese, crumbled
- 1 tablespoons olive oil
- 1 tablespoons red wine vinegar
- 1 teaspoon dried thyme
- 1 teaspoon dried oregano
- Sea salt and black pepper, to taste

STEPS

Mix every one of the ingredients in a container.
You can eat right away or marinate in the refrigerator thirty minutes before eating, so the flavors have time to meld well,
Serve, as you can see in the picture, with cheese, c, rackers, Serrano ham, or your favorite accompaniment.

Banana Nut Muffins 100% Whole Grain

Ingredients

- 1 $\frac{1}{2}$ cups walnuts, toasted and chopped
- 5 tablespoons canola or walnut oil
- 1 tablespoon walnut oil (substitute canola oil if you don't have any)
- $\frac{1}{2}$ cup brown sugar
- 1 egg
- $\frac{1}{2}$ cup nonfat Greek yogurt (plain, unsweetened)
- 5 ripe bananas, mashed
- 1$\frac{1}{2}$ cups wholemeal
- 1 $\frac{1}{2}$ teaspoon of baking powder
- $\frac{1}{2}$ teaspoon of salt

STEPS

Preheat oven to 350°F / 180°C.
Prepare 18 paper cups (4 cm diameter) and place them in the muffin or cupcake tray. You can also use silicone muffin tins.
When the oven temperature reaches 350°F, place the pecans on a baking sheet and toast in the oven for 5 minutes. Remove from the oven and chop them.
In a medium bowl, mix canola oil, walnut oil, brown sugar, egg, and yogurt. Whisk to combine, then add the mashed banana and chopped toasted walnuts.
Add the flour, baking powder, and salt.

Add $\frac{1}{4}$ cup of the mixture (use a measuring cup) to each paper or silicone cup to fill all 18 cups.
Bake for 23 to 25 minutes, or until the tops of muffins are nicely browned.
Cool.

Hummus

Ingredients for two bowls:

- 6 ounces (175 g) of dried chickpeas
- 1 tablespoon + 1 small pinch of baking soda
- 2 ounces (70 g) of tahini (sesame paste)
- juice of 1 lemon
- 1 to 2 garlic cloves
- ½ teaspoon ground cumin
- Salt to taste
- Olive oil
- Fresh parsley (per serving)

STEPS

Soak dried chickpeas in room temperature water with one tablespoon of baking soda for 12 hours (overnight).
Drain, rinse, soak again in clean water for about 4 hours.
Drain, rinse and add enough cold water to cover 2 cm above the chickpeas. Add a small pinch of baking soda.
Bring to a boil and cook for 1-1.5 hours until the chickpeas are tender and easy to puree.
Drain the cooked chickpeas and reserve the cooking water. Reserve a handful of whole chickpeas (for decoration)
Puree the rest of the chickpeas in a food processor. Add a little cooking water if necessary to give it a pure consistency. Let cool for 15 -20 minutes.
Add tahini, lemon juice and garlic (if using), ground cumin, salt, and one tablespoon olive oil.
Blend again in a food processor until smooth. Add cooking water to give it the desired consistency. This should be thick, so it is easy to pick up with a piece of bread but soft and spreadable.

Pita With Eggs And Vegetables

Ingredients

- 15ml/1tbsp vegetable oil (preferably 100% canola oil)
- 2 sliced spring onions
- 3,5 ounces (100g) cherry tomatoes cut in half or Tomatoes cut into cubes
- 4 large eggs
- 2 toasted whole wheat pita bread

STEPS

Heat the oil in a nonstick skillet, add the onion and tomatoes, fry for 1 minute.
Beat eggs and salt and pepper (ideally freshly ground). Add eggs to the pan and simmer for 3 minutes. Stir completely and reserve.
Cut the pita bread in half and fill it with the preparation. Serve hot.

Egg And Mushrooms On Toast

Ingredients

- Olive oil 30ml/2 tablespoons
- Sliced Portobello Mushrooms 8 ounces (225g)
- A dash of Worcestershire sauce to taste
- Salt and freshly ground black pepper
- 4 large eggs
- 4 slices whole-grain seedless bread, toasted
- A handful of chopped parsley (optional)

STEPS

Heat half the oil in a non-stick frying pan Add the mushrooms and cook over high heat for 3-4 minutes or until tender.
Add the Worcestershire sauce and season to taste.
Transfer to a container and keep warm. Wipe the pan, add the remaining oil and gently break eggs. Cook over medium heat for about 3 minutes, using a spoon to pour the hot oil over the egg yolks until the eggs are cooked to your liking.
Divide the toasts among four plates, add the mushrooms on top together with the parsley and the fried eggs. Serve immediately.

Baked Eggs

Ingredients

- 1 cup washed raw quinoa
- 4 whites
- 4 eggs
- 20 stalks of green asparagus cooked and chopped
- 6 ounces (180 grams) of chopped zucchini
- 1 red pepper, chopped
- 3 cloves garlic, minced
- 1 teaspoon of fine herbs
- 2 teaspoons
- Balsamic vinegar
- 1 tablespoon olive oil
- Cooking spray
- Salt and pepper
- To decorate: ½ ounces (15 grams) of Parmesan, parsley sprigs

STEPS

Preheat the oven to medium temperature 180 ° C / 356 ° F for 20 minutes; Cook quinoa until it grains.
Mix the vegetables with quinoa. Season with vinegar, olive oil, garlic, and herbs fine. Salpimiente. Beat egg whites and stir the mixture. Pour the mixture on a refractory plate greased with cooking spray.
Make four holes in the mixture and break an egg into each. Take the oven for 30 minutes or until or curdle. Garnish with Parmesan cheese and parsley branches.

Chickpea Egg Bowl

Ingredients

- 2 Boiled Eggs, Large & Chopped
- 2 Tablespoons Parsley, Fresh & Chopped Fine
- 1 Green Onion, Chopped Fine
- 1 Tablespoon Lemon Juice, Fresh
- 1 Cup Chickpeas, Rinsed & Drained

STEPS

Add your chickpeas and 1 ½ cups of water into your instant pot, and then stir in your ingredients. Make sure it's mixed well, and then cook on high pressure for 12 minutes. Allow the ingredients to cook and quick release, and then mix in your remaining ingredients. Serve warm.

Fresh Cheese with Tomato

Ingredients

- ¼ Teaspoon Red Wine Vinegar
- 2 Tomatoes, Chopped
- 1 Tablespoon Olive Oil
- ¼ Cup Cottage Cheese
- Sea Salt & Black Pepper to Taste

STEPS

Add your tomatoes in a blender and puree until smooth.
Add in your remaining ingredients except for the oil, and blend to make it smooth.
Take your instant pot and press sauté. Once it's hot, add in your oil.
Add your tomato mix in, and cook for three to four minutes.
Add them to the Cooking pot, and combine well. Serve warm.

Broccoli & Eggs

Ingredients

- 1 Onion, Chopped
- 6 Eggs, Beaten
- 1 Tablespoon All Purpose Flour
- 16 onces (450g) Broccoli, Chopped into Florets

STEPS

Mix your eggs, spices and flour in a mixing bowl and then add in your broccoli. Toss to coat, and then set it to the side.
Line a baking pan with parchment paper and grease it with Cooking spray. Add in your broccoli.
Pour a cup of water into the instant pot, and then add in your steamer basket.
Arrange your pan in the basket, and then close the lid.
Cook on high pressure for thirty minutes, and then quick release.
Serve warm.

Garlic Eggs

Ingredients

- 1 Tablespoon Olive Oil
- 6 Tomatoes, Small
- 4 Eggs
- 1 Teaspoon Garlic, Minced
- 1 Teaspoon Turmeric Powder
- 1 Green Onion, Chopped
- Sea Salt & Black Pepper to Taste

STEPS

Halve your tomatoes, and then set them to the side.
Place a tablespoon of olive oil into your instant pot and press sauté before adding your tomatoes. Put the cut side down, and then add in your garlic and turmeric.
Add in your eggs, and stir them with a spatula to scramble. Season with salt and pepper.
Cook for about 15 minutes, and sprinkle with chopped green onion to serve.

Banana Quinoa

Ingredients

- ¾ Cup Quinoa, Soaked in Water for 1 Hour
- 8 Ounces (240 ml) Almond Milk, Canned
- ¾ Cup Water
- 1 Teaspoon Vanilla Extract, pure
- ½ Cup Banana, Peeled & Sliced
- A Pinch of Sea Salt

Topping
- 6 Banana Slices
- Chocolate, Grated (Optional)

STEPS

Add all your quinoa ingredients to the instant pot and secure the lid. Press rice, and then cook for twelve minutes on low pressure. Release the pressure naturally and then stir. Place in serving bowls and top with banana and chocolate.

Almond Risotto

Ingredients

- 2 Cups Almond Milk, Vanilla
- 2 Tablespoons Honey, Raw
- 1 Teaspoon Vanilla Extract, Pure
- ¼ Cup Almond Flakes, Toasted for Garnish
- ½ Cup Arborio Rice

STEPS

Place all of your ingredients into the instant pot, and then cook on high pressure for five minutes.
Allow for a natural pressure release and serve garnished with almond flakes.

Coconut Risotto

Ingredients

- 2 Cups Coconut Milk
- ½ Cup Arborio Rice
- 2 Tablespoons Coconut Sugar
- 1 Teaspoon Vanilla Extract
- ¼ Cup Coconut Flakes, Toasted for Garnish

STEPS

Throw all of your ingredients into the instant pot and then cook on high pressure for five minutes.
Allow for a natural pressure release for twenty minutes before serving with coconut flakes.

Breakfast Quinoa

Ingredients

- 1 Cup Quinoa, Rinsed & Drained
- 3 Cups Almond Milk, Vanilla
- ¼ Cup Almonds
- 1 Cup Blackberries, Chopped
- ¼ Teaspoon Cinnamon

STEPS

Start by placing your quinoa in your instant pot, and then pour in your milk. Add in your cinnamon. Seal your instant pot before setting it to manual settings.
Cook at high pressure for two minutes before allowing for a natural pressure release. Top with almonds and berries before serving.

Coconut Yogurt

Ingredients

- 1 Tablespoon Gelatin
- 3 Cups Coconut Cream
- 1 Package Yogurt Starter

STEPS

Start by adding in your coconut cream to your instant pot before pressing the yogurt setting.
Remove the pot and turn it off.
Allow it to cool in the fridge for ten minutes before moving onto the next step.
Afterwards, stir in your yogurt starter until it's smooth, and put your pot back into your instant pot.
Press your yogurt button again, setting the time to eight hours. Stir in your gelatin gradually.
Refrigerate for at least four hours before serving.

Squash & Apple Porridge

Ingredients

- 1 Delicate Squash, Peeled
- 4 Apples, Cored & Sliced
- 1/8 Teaspoon Ground Ginger
- 1/2 Teaspoon Cinnamon
- 2 Tablespoons Maple Syrup

STEPS

Start by placing your apples and squash in your instant pot before adding in a cup of water.
Sprinkle with ginger, a dash of salt and cinnamon before sealing your pot and setting it to manual. Cook on high pressure for eight minutes.
Allow for a natural pressure release and then slice the squash.
Transfer your squash and everything else in a blender, pulsing until smooth.
Drizzle with maple syrup before serving.

Refreshing Mango and Pear Smoothie

Ingredients

- 1 ripe mango, cored and chopped
- 1/2 mango, peeled, pitted and chopped
- 1 cup kale, chopped
- 1/2 cup plain Greek yogurt
- 2 ice cubes

STEPS

Add pear, mango, yogurt, kale, and mango to a blender and puree.
Add ice and blend until you have a smooth texture.
Serve and enjoy!

Barley Porridge

Ingredients

- 1 cup barley
- 1 cup wheat berries
- 2 cups unsweetened almond milk
- 2 cups water
- Toppings such as hazelnuts, honey, berry, etc.

STEPS

Take a medium saucepan and place it over medium-high heat
Place barley, almond milk, wheat berries, water and bring to a boil.
Lower down heat to low and simmer for 25 minutes.
Divide amongst serving bowls and top with your desired toppings.
Serve and enjoy!

Strawberry and Rhubarb Smoothie

Ingredients

- 1 rhubarb stalk, chopped
- 1 cup fresh strawberries, sliced
- ½ cup plain Greek strawberries
- A Pinch of ground cinnamon
- 3 ice cubes

STEPS

Take a small saucepan and fill with water over high heat.
Bring to boil and add rhubarb, boil for 3 minutes.
Drain and transfer to a blender
Add strawberries, honey, yogurt, cinnamon and pulse mixture until smooth.
Add ice cubes and blend until thick and has no lumps.
Pour into glass and enjoy chilled.

Cheesy Zucchini Omelette

Ingredients

- 4 large eggs
- 2-3 medium zucchinis
- 1-2 garlic cloves, crushed
- 4 tablespoon grated cheese
- Season as needed

STEPS

Take a bowl and add grated zucchinis, make sure to peel as the skin is bitter.
Take a bowl and break in eggs a, crushed garlic and cheese.
Pour the mixture in a hot frying pan with a little bit of oil and place it over medium heat, keep a lid on.
Once the egg is cooked nicely, and the bottom is crispy and golden, serve an enjoy with a garnish of chopped parsley.
Enjoy!

Easy to Munch Olive Cherry and Olive Bites

Ingredients

- 24 cherry tomatoes, halved
- 24 black olives, pitted
- 24 feta cheese cubes
- 24 toothpick/decorative skewers

STEPS

Use a toothpick or skewer and thread feta cheese, black olives, cherry tomato halves in that order.
Repeat until all the ingredients are used.
Arrange in a serving platter.
Serve and enjoy!

Power Packed Oatmeal

Ingredients

- 1/4 cup quick Cooking oats
- 1/4 cup milk
- 2 tablespoons Greek yogurt
- 1/4 banana, mashed
- 2 1/4 tablespoons flaxseed meal

STEPS

Whisk in all of the ingredients in a bowl.
Transfer the bowl to your fridge and let it refrigerate for 15 minutes.
Serve and enjoy!

Banana Steel Oats

Ingredients

- 1 small banana
- 1 cup almond milk
- 1/4 teaspoon cinnamon, ground
- 1/2 cup rolled oats
- 1 tablespoon honey

STEPS

Take a saucepan and add half the banana, whisk in almond milk, ground cinnamon.
Season with salt.
Stir until the banana is mashed well, bring the mixture to a boil and stir in oats.
Lower heat to medium-low and simmer for 5-7 minutes until the oats are tender.
Dice remaining half of banana and top oatmeal.
Enjoy!

Hearty Pumpkin Oats

Ingredients

- 1 cup quick-Cooking rolled oats
- 3/4 cup milk
- 1/2 cup canned pumpkin puree
- 1/4 teaspoon pumpkin pie spice
- 1 teaspoon ground cinnamon

STEPS

Take a safe microwave bowl and add oats, milk, and microwave on high for 1-2 minutes.

Add more milk if needed to achieve your desired consistency.
Cook for 30 seconds more.
Stir in pumpkin puree, pumpkin pie spice, ground cinnamon.
Heat gently and enjoy!

Cool Red Pepper and Olive Omelette

Ingredients

- 4 large eggs
- ¾ cup feta cheese, roughly chopped
- 2 red peppers
- 1 onion, chopped
- 12 black olives, stoned and halved

STEPS

Take a frying pan and add onions and pepper, place it over medium heat and sweat for 10 minutes (lid on).
Take a bowl and beat eggs lightly, add feta cheese, olives and season with salt and pepper.
Add the mixture to the pan and tilt until the veggies are covered.
Place lid again and fry on medium heat until the egg mixture starts to become solid, if you feel like it, flip the Omelette, otherwise, let it cool until the bottom shows a crispy golden texture.
Serve with a garnish of fresh chopped parsley.

Avocado and Blueberry Medley

Ingredients

- 1 frozen banana
- 2 avocados, quartered
- 2 cups berries
- Maple syrup as needed

STEPS

Take your blender and add all ingredients except maple syrup.
Add ice water and blend.
Garnish with syrup and pour in smoothie glasses. Enjoy!

Herbed Parmesan Walnuts

Ingredients

- ½ cup Parmigiano-Reggiano cheese
- ½ teaspoon Italian herb seasoning and garlic salt
- 1 teaspoon parsley flakes
- 2 cups walnuts
- 1 egg white

STEPS

Pre-heat your oven to 250 degrees F° /120°C.
Take a bowl and add all ingredients except egg white and walnuts.
Whisk in egg and stir in halved walnuts and mix well.
Transfer the mixture to greased baking sheet and bake for 30 minutes.

CHAPTER 6

Lunch

Nutrition and food have always represented the fundamental pillars of the life and culture of people. However, in recent decades, changes in these habits have been noted. Such transformations in nutrition patterns and, above all, lifestyle influence the population's health.

The Mediterranean diet is a food model endorsed by the World Health Organization (WHO) and the Food and Agriculture Organization of the United Nations (FAO). It is characterized by different foods: olive oil as the main fat, vegetables, fruits and vegetables, legumes, nuts, cheeses and yogurt, fish, bread, and wheat derivatives, and moderate consumption of wine and meat. The Mediterranean dietary pattern that comes from the interaction between peoples for centuries is also related to regular physical activity. This evidence shows the beneficial effects of the Mediterranean diet on health.

However, in recent decades, Mediterranean countries have experienced profound globalization, which directly impacts dietary patterns and compromises the cultural and health heritage that the traditional Mediterranean diet represents.

Mediterranean Diet Threats

The new lifestyle, together with the demographic and sociological changes that have occurred, translates into:
• Less time to cook,
• Lunches away from home,
• Supermarkets that offer products out of season,
• Unhealthy and high-calorie food offered by fast-food chains,
• Reduced physical activity

The fact of reducing the consumption of fruits, vegetables, cereals, and legumes, and betting on the increase in calories from meat, fats, and sugars added to food as well as the excessive use of salt, leads to the gradual abandonment of traditional eating habits and the appearance of diseases related to the new lifestyles acquired that translate into unhealthy habits.

It should not be forgotten that acquiring and promoting adequate eating habits are very important from an early age. At that age, the basic pillars for maintaining this lifestyle are established even in adulthood. Betting on a Mediterranean diet means:

- Enjoy its nutritional qualities,
- Stimulate local production and consumption,
- Lower prevalence and incidence of cardiovascular diseases in Mediterranean countries,
- Lower rate of obesity and longer life expectancy,
- Encourage an active lifestyle.

In short, the Mediterranean diet represents a stamp of authenticity, quality, and health and is of great importance in the current context of globalization of markets.

Did you know that Mediterranean food has been declared Cultural Heritage of Humanity? And, of course, we understand why! With the rich flavors so characteristic of that area, they deserve that and many other distinctions. One of its most delicious qualities is the use of fresh fish and ingredients, which is why its salads are an out-of-this-world flavor experience. Although, of course, their dishes for dinner and desserts are not far behind.

Recipes

Hot Spinach And Artichoke Cups

Ingredients

- 24 wonton sheets one can (14 oz.) artichoke hearts, drained, finely chopped
- 1 cup KRAFT Shredded Mozzarella Cheese one pkg. (10 oz.) frozen chopped spinach, thawed and well-drained
- 1/3 cup KRAFT Mayo with Olive Oil Reduced Fat Mayonnaise
- 1/3 cup grated KRAFT Grated Parmesan Cheese
- 1/4 cup finely chopped red bell pepper two garlic cloves, finely minced

STEPS

Heat oven to 350°F / 175°C.
Place one wonton wrapper in each of 24 small muffin cups, sprayed with cooking spray; let the edges of the sheets exceed the top of the cup. Bake for 5 min. Meanwhile, mix the remaining ingredients.
Put the artichoke mixture in the wonton cups.
Bake cups 12 to 14 min. or until filling is heated through and rims of cups are golden brown.

Salad With Chickpeas, Bulgur, And Orange

Ingredients

- 1 ½ cups of water
- ½ cup bulgur wheat, uncooked
- 6 cups of chopped romaine lettuce two oranges, peeled, cut in half lengthwise and into ¼ -inch slices breadthways six green onions (chives), sliced
- ½ cup KRAFT Balsamic Vinaigrette Dressing

STEPS

Bring water to a boil in a small saucepan; incorporate the bulgur. Put the lid on; simmer for 15 min. on the medium-low boil. Or until water is absorbed. Let bulgur cool, uncovered, 20 min.
Combine the rest of the ingredients in a large bowl.
Add the bulgur; mix it up a bit.

How to serve:

Top with ½ cup ATHENOS Crumbled Feta Cheese before serving in your favorite flavor.

Bruschetta With Balsamic Dressing, Olives, And Pepper

Ingredients

- ¼ cup KRAFT Balsamic Vinaigrette Dressing two garlic cloves, finely minced one green, one red, and one yellow bell pepper cut into thin strips
- ¼ cup of water
- 12 slices (1/4-inch thick) baguette
- ¾ cup pitted green olives one tablespoon capers two tablespoons chopped Italian (flat) parsley

STEPS

Heat oven to 425°F / 220°C.
Heat dressing over medium heat in a large skillet. Add garlic; cook and stir for 1 min. Add the peppers and water. Let all this boil; cover the skillet. Cook it over low heat, maintaining a gentle boil for 20 min. Or until peppers are tender; remember to stir from time to time.
Meanwhile, arrange bread slices in a single layer on a baking sheet. Bake for 10 min. or until well browned.
Add olives and capers to the pepper mixture; cook and stir one min. or until everything is heated. Spoon mixture over toasted slices; sprinkle with parsley.

How to prepare the peppers:
To prepare the peppers, wash them well and remove the core. Scoop out the seeds and membranes. Wrap the cut pieces tightly in plastic wrap and refrigerate to preserve their fresh flavor and crisp texture.

Mediterranean Marinated Vegetable Salad

Ingredients

- 2 large tomatoes, cut into wedges,
- 1 green and one yellow bell pepper, coarsely chopped
- 1 zucchini cut in half lengthwise, and sliced
- ¼ cup red onion cut into wedges
- ½ cup KRAFT Zesty Italian Dressing two tablespoons chopped fresh basil leaves two garlic cloves, finely minced
- 1 cup KRAFT Natural Three Cheese Crumbles

STEPS

Combine the tomatoes and vegetables in a large salad bowl.
Combine dressing, basil, and garlic. Pour this over vegetable mixture; toss to coat.
Add cheese; mix lightly. Refrigerate the salad for 1 hour.

Prepare with KRAFT Lite Zesty Italian Reduced Fat Dressing. The salad can be stored in the refrigerator for up to 24 hours before serving.
Just before serving, top with chopped cooked chicken.

Mediterranean Cheese

Ingredients

- 1 pkg. (8 oz.) PHILADELPHIA Cream Cheese softened
- 1 jar (7 oz), roasted red bell peppers, drained and chopped
- 1 pkg. (4 oz.) ATHENOS Traditional Feta Cheese
- ½ cup chopped Kalamata olives (about 40)
- 1/4 cup KRAFT Balsamic Vinaigrette Dressing
- 2 tablespoons chopped fresh parsley

STEPS

Spread the cream cheese on the bottom of a plate or pie pan.
Mix remaining ingredients; top with cream cheese.
Serve cheese spread with RITZ Crackers.
Prepare with KRAFT Greek Vinaigrette Dressing.

Zucchini And Aubergines Stuffed With Tomato And Cheese

Ingredients
- 1 cup red, orange, and yellow cherry tomatoes mixed, chopped
- ½ cup KRAFT Tuscan House Italian Dressing, divided
- 2 small zucchini and 2 Chinese eggplants, ends trimmed
- 1 ½ cups KRAFT Finely Shredded Italian* Five Cheese Blend
- 2 tablespoons chopped fresh basil

STEPS

Heat oiled grill to medium heat.
Toss tomatoes with two tablespoons of the dressing.
Cut zucchini and eggplant in halves lengthwise; brush with 2 tbsp, Of the remaining dressing. Grill cut side up for 12 minutes or until tender, turning after six minutes. And brushing with remaining dressing. Put the cut faces back up. Top with cheese; broil one min. or until melted. Transfer them to a platter.
Add the basil to the tomato mixture and stir lightly. Spoon this mixture over the roasted greens (vegetables) and cut it half.

Shrimp Bruschetta With Orzo Pasta

Ingredients

- 1 ¼ cups orzo pasta, uncooked
- ¾ cup Italian Vinaigrette Dressing made with Extra Virgin Olive Oil KRAFT Italian Vinaigrette Dressing made with Extra Virgin Olive Oil, divided three cloves garlic, finely minced, divided
- 1 pound raw large shrimp, peeled and deveined
- 1 ½ pounds cherry tomatoes (about 40), divided
- ½ pound (90 g) French bread (half a 16-oz loaf), cut into 24 cubes one bunch of green onions (about 8)
- 1 cup fresh basil leaves, chopped
- ¼ cup grated KRAFT Grated Parmesan Cheese

STEPS

Heat grill to medium heat.
Cook the pasta as directed on the package. Meanwhile, mix 1/4 cup of the dressing and 1/3 of the garlic. Thread shrimp onto six skewers; thread 24 tomatoes onto six additional skewers, alternating with bread cubes. Grill all skewers for three min., turning and occasionally basting with half of the dressing mixture. Remove the tomato skewers from the grill. Arrange the onions in a single layer on the grill. Grill onions and shrimp for 2 to 3 minutes or until shrimp turn pink and onions are crisp-tender; remember to brush with the remaining dressing mixture occasionally.
Drain pasta; put it in a large bowl. Cut the remaining tomatoes into quarters. Add to pasta and remaining dressing, garlic, and basil; mix everything lightly. Slice onions; stir into pasta mixture. Sprinkle the pasta with Parmesan. Serve it with the shrimp skewers.

Caesar Salad With Romaine Lettuce And Grilled Chicken

Ingredients

- 2 heads romaine lettuce, cut in half lengthwise one tablespoon of olive oil, divided into four small boneless skinless chicken breasts (1 lb.)
- 2 cups grape tomatoes, cut in half
- ½ cup croutons (croutons)
- ¼ cup finely sliced red onion
- ¼ cup pitted Kalamata olives
- ¼ cup grated KRAFT Grated Parmesan Cheese
- 1/2 cup KRAFT Classic Caesar Dressing

STEPS

Heat grill to medium-high heat.
Brush the lettuce evenly with half the oil, then brush the chicken with the remaining oil.
Grill chicken for 6 to 8 min. on each side or until done (internal temperature of 165°F/80°C). Transfer to a cutting board and let rest for 5 min.
Meanwhile, place lettuce, cut sides down, on the grill rack. Grill 3 to 4 min. or until light marks on both sides, turning after 2 min. of cooking.
Slice the chicken and place it on a platter. Add lettuce and remaining ingredients except cheese and dressing. Sprinkle with cheese and drizzle with dressing.
Grill a boneless beef steak, such as a flank or sirloin, to medium doneness (internal temperature of 160°F/80°C). Use this steak instead of the chicken.
Chop the roasted lettuce halves before placing them on the platter.
Prepare the recipe with KRAFT Shredded Parmesan Cheese.

Spanish paella

Ingredients

- 1 ½ cups reduced-sodium fat-free chicken broth
- 1/8 teaspoon of saffron threads

- ½ pound (90 g) Iberian chorizo, cut into ½-inch slices
- three slices OSCAR MAYER Bacon Bacon, cut into 1-inch pieces
- one can (14.5 oz) diced tomatoes, drained
- one red bell pepper, chopped
- ½ cup chopped onion four garlic cloves, finely minced
- ¼ cup KRAFT Zesty Italian Dressing
- 1 cup long-grain white rice, uncooked
- ¾ pound medium shrimp, raw, peeled (with tails on), deveined
- 1 pound tilapia filets, cut into 1-inch pieces
- ½ pound mussels, well washed, without beards
- ¼ cup frozen peas, thawed

STEPS

Heat oven to 325°F/ 160°C.
Cook the broth and saffron threads in a small saucepan over medium heat until they come to a gentle boil.
Meanwhile, cook and stir sausage and bacon in a large ovenproof skillet on medium heat for 4 to 5 min. or until ready. Remove meat from skillet with a slotted spoon; drain on a paper towel.
Add tomatoes, bell pepper, onion, garlic, and dressing to fat in skillet; cook and stir for 5 min. Stir in bouillon mixture; let it boil gently. Add the rice, meat, shrimp, and tilapia; stir everything. Top with mussels, nestling them in the rice mixture; cover skillet.
Bake the paella for 25 to 30 min. or until liquid is absorbed and mussels open. Discard unopened mussels. Cover the paella with the peas.

Grilled Chicken With Fresh Spinach And Tomato Confit

Ingredients (4 diners)

- 4 small chicken breasts
- 1 thick slice of fresh ginger
- 2 cloves of garlic
- 14 ounces (400 grams) of spinach sprouts
- 2-3 tablespoons of soy sauce
- 1 teaspoon of salt
- 1 teaspoon extra virgin olive oil
- 25-30 candied cherry tomatoes (see recipe)
- 1 ounces (30 grams) of feta cheese
- a handful of toasted pistachios
- freshly ground black pepper

STEPS

Clean the chicken breasts off the skin and the possible fat that they may have, dry them well with absorbent kitchen paper. Heat a large skillet with a little extra virgin olive oil, salt the chicken breasts on both sides, and place them in the skillet over medium-high heat to cook until golden brown.
Meanwhile, peel and finely chop the fresh ginger (grate it if you prefer) and the garlic cloves. Prepare the fresh spinach shoots to sauté them for a few seconds in the pan. When the chicken breasts are almost ready, add the garlic and ginger, give them a couple of turns and add the spinach and soy sauce; stir so that the spinach loses some of its water and volume, and remove from the heat.

Keep the candied tomatoes out of the fridge for a while before they are too cold. Crumble the feta cheese for serving and peel the toasted pistachios.

Serve the chicken breast on flat plates on a bed of spinach sprouts. Next, spread out the candied cherry tomatoes, crumbled feta cheese, pistachios, and freshly ground black pepper. Finish with a tablespoon of tomato confit oil.

Chicken With Spinach And Lemon Cream

Ingredients

- 4 small chicken breasts
- 4 radishes
- freshly ground black pepper
- grated lemon peel
- Maldon salt
- extra virgin olive oil.
- For the spinach and lemon cream
- 10 ounces (300 grams) of fresh spinach
- 1 shallot
- 10 ounces (250-300 grams) of unsweetened almond milk
- the grated skin of a lemon
- 1 tsp lemongrass powder
- freshly ground black pepper
- a pinch of salt
- 1 tsp of honey (optional).

STEPS

Start by preparing the spinach cream, put them in a low saucepan or a large skillet with the finely chopped shallot, almond milk, grated lemon peel, and lemongrass the pepper, and salt to taste.

Take it to the fire, and as soon as the almond drink is hot, start stirring so that the spinach loses volume; it will be easier to cook them and that all the ingredients mix well. Cook over low heat for about five minutes; without letting the liquid evaporate, you can partially cover the pan to avoid it and favor the cooking of the vegetables.

Transfer the spinach with the almond milk to the blender glass and blend until you obtain a fine and homogeneous cream. If it is too light, you can add a pinch of xanthan, it is a good resource (but it is not essential at all) for these cases, and it does not modify the flavor. But you have to put very little, approximately the tip of a knife, all depending on the desired density, but it must be a light cream.

Try the cream to rectify salt, spices... and if it is a bit strong or astringent on the palate due to the brief cooking of the spinach, you can add a pinch of honey. Reserve hot while you prepare the chicken.

In a frying pan or skillet greased with extra virgin olive oil, cook the chicken breasts over medium heat to brown on the outside and cook on the inside. While the chicken is cooking, you can prepare the radishes, wash them, cut off the tip and laminate them with a hand mandolin.

Pour the cream as a base on the plate; there should not be too much, as it acts as a sauce for the meat. Place the chicken breast on the spinach and lemon cream and add Maldon salt, freshly ground black pepper, and grated lemon peel. Place two mounds of sliced radish and finish with a few extra virgin olive oil drops. Bon Appetit!

Chicken Breast With Fennel Salad

Ingredients

For the chicken
- 4 small chicken breasts
- 1 tablespoon extra virgin olive oil
- A pinch of salt
- 1 teaspoon smoked paprika flakes
- one bag of canons.

For the fennel salad
- 250 grams of fennel bulb (1 piece)
- 2-3 sprigs of fresh coriander
- ½ tsp pepper-lemon
- ½ tsp of smoked Vera paprika flakes.

For the vinaigrette
- 1 ounces (30 ml) extra virgin olive oil
- 0,3 ounces (10 ml) sesame oil
- 0,3 ounces (10 ml) Sherry vinegar
- A pinch of salt.

STEPS

For the chicken

Clean the chicken breasts by squaring them and drying them with absorbent paper. Heat a griddle or grill with a little extra virgin olive oil, and when hot, add the chicken. Add salt to taste and cook over medium-high heat so that it browns on the outside and cooks on the inside. It is normal for chicken made in this way to be juicy in the thickest part and somewhat drier in the thinnest part.

For the fennel salad

Meanwhile, prepare the fennel salad; first, cut four slices and cook them together with the chicken on the grill with a little extra virgin olive oil. Cut the rest of the fennel into julienne strips and put it in a bowl; wash and dry the coriander and chop it, add it to the bowl, and season with the pepper-lemon (mixture of spices) the smoked paprika flakes.

For the vinaigrette

Prepare the vinaigrette by mixing the two oils, the Sherry vinegar, and the salt. Shake well and dress the fennel salad, reserving a little for the plating. Finally, wash and drain the lamb's lettuce very well; if you wish, you can cut the base of the bunches of leaves.

Arrange the lamb's lettuce on flat plates and then place the chicken breast, serve the grilled fennel on one side and place the fennel salad on top of the meat. Finish dressing with a little more vinaigrette and eat.

Grilled Chicken With Chanterelles And Pumpkin

Ingredients

- 14 ounces (400 grams) butternut squash, peeled and seeded
- 14 ounces (400 grams) of chanterelles
- four cloves of garlic
- a pinch of black pepper
- a pinch of allspice
- ½ tsp of ground ñora
- A pinch of salt
- 1 tablespoon extra virgin olive oil
- four small chicken breasts
- ½ bunch of chives

STEPS

Cut the butternut squash into cubes, clean the chanterelles to remove any dirt they may have and chop them, peel the garlic cloves, and cut them into slices.

Heat a large frying pan with a little extra virgin olive oil over medium heat, add the pumpkin with a little salt and sauté it. When golden and slightly tender, add the chanterelles and garlic cloves, and sauté over medium-high heat.

Season with black pepper, allspice, ground ñora, and salt, and add extra virgin olive oil if necessary.

While the mushrooms are made with the pumpkin, cook the chicken skillet on medium-high heat, seasoned to taste, and with a trickle of extra virgin olive oil in another pan or skillet. Play with the temperature to get the chicken to be golden, slightly toasted, with a juicy interior, but well done.

Serve each chicken breast on its plate, accompanied by the garnish of chanterelles and pumpkin. Optionally, you can add a few grains of pomegranate. Finely chop the fresh chives and spread them over the plates. Add a little Maldon salt and a dash of extra virgin olive oil.

Chicken With Tomato Compote And Cornicabra

Ingredients

- 4 chicken breasts
- 1 tablespoon extra virgin olive oil
- a pinch of fine salt

For the tomato and cornicabra compote

- 17 $\frac{1}{2}$ ounces (500 grams) of ripe tomato (peeled)
- $\frac{1}{2}$ tsp of sugar
- 1 tsp of salt
- four basil leaves
- one sprig of rosemary
- w/ black pepper
- $\frac{1}{2}$ tsp sweet paprika
- $\frac{1}{2}$ c/c of seven spices
- 1 tablespoon of soy sauce
- 3-4 tablespoons of cornicabra variety extra virgin olive oil.

STEPS

Wash the tomatoes, cut them in half, grate them, and put them in a saucepan with sugar and salt. Put the saucepan on the fire and cook over medium-high heat until it reduces by half; stir from time to time.

When you have reduced by half, you will still have vegetation water, you will have to continue reducing, but it is time to incorporate the basil, rosemary, and spices. Continue with the cooking, lower the heat to continue with the reduction without splashing the tomato, and for the aromas to merge gently.

Reduce the tomato until obtaining a compote, then remove the saucepan from the heat (and remove the sprig of rosemary, you can remove the basil if you wish), add the soy sauce and the cornicabra extra virgin olive oil, mix well, the sauce of tomato will acquire brightness and body, try it in case it is necessary to rectify it. Booking.

Put a pan with a thread of extra virgin olive oil to heat to make the chicken breasts; as they are made whole and are thick, it is convenient to put the temperature on medium or medium-high heat so that it browns slowly on the outside and cook inside. Salt the chicken breasts to taste. Serve a thick string of tomato compote at the base of the dish; it must be hot, and place the freshly cooked chicken breast on top. Decorate with some fresh basil leaves, drop a few flakes of salt and prepare a good homemade bread to accompany.

Chicken Breast With Parsnip And Rosemary Sauce

Ingredients

- four chicken breasts
- 10 ounces (280 grams) of parsnips
- 3 ounces (75 grams) of red onion
- 3 garlic cloves
- ½ tsp five freshly ground peppers
- one sprig of rosemary
- Salt
- 1 tablespoon of extra virgin olive oil
- 14 ounces (400 grams) of ham broth
- 2 ounces (60 grams) of cream cheese
- Salt Maldon.

STEPS

Clean the chicken breasts leaving them without skin or fat. Reserve in the refrigerator well covered while you prepare the sauce.
Peel the parsnips into thin slices; cut the widest part half. Peel and finely chop the onion; peel the garlic and cut it into slices. Heat a wide, deep frying pan with a fund of extra virgin olive oil; when it is hot, add the garlic, give it a couple of turns, and then add the parsnip, the onion, a little mixture of five freshly ground peppers, the sprig of rosemary and a pinch of salt.

Sauté over medium-low heat for about ten minutes or until they begin to soften. Next, add the ham broth and let it come to a boil. First, raise the heat, lower it again, and cook for 10-12 minutes without covering the pan. Once the parsnips are cooked, transfer them to the blender container with the broth and add the cream cheese, the leaves of the sprig of rosemary, a drizzle of extra virgin olive oil, and truffle oil. Blend until you get a creamy, fine, and shiny sauce. Reserve hot. To make the chicken breasts, heat a griddle or frying pan with a little extra virgin olive oil and cook the chicken over medium heat so that the heat reaches the center of the meat and cooks it while browning the surface on both sides. Season the breasts to taste.
Serve two or three generous tablespoons of a parsnip, rosemary, and truffle sauce as a base on the plate, making a tear. Cut the chicken breast into wide slices for presentation, and place them on top of the sauce. Season with a mixture of five peppers, a thread of extra virgin olive oil, and Maldon salt. Garnish with a sprig of fresh rosemary.

Grilled Chicken With Bimi, Soy Sauce And Kimchi

Ingredients

- 14 ounces (400 grams) bimini
- 4 tbsp frozen sweet corn (or canned, but no added sugar)
- 2-3 cloves of garlic
- 4 small chicken breasts
- 1 tbsp of extra virgin olive oil
- 1 tbsp of sesame seeds

- a pinch of salt.

For the sauce
- 2 tbsp.(30 grams) of soy sauce
- 1 tbsp. (10 grams) of kimchi sauce
- 1/5 tbsp. (8 grams)of sesame oil
- 1 tbsp. (10 grams)of extra virgin olive oil
- 1 tsp of toasted sesame seeds.

STEPS

Clean the time and steam it in the container you usually use. If you want to do it faster, you can boil it briefly, but without submerging it completely in water, heat a large pan with less than an inch of water, cover it and bring it to a boil. Let cook for about 5 minutes, then uncover and let the water evaporate.

Put the grill (you can also do it on a griddle or in the same pan) to heat with a little extra virgin olive oil and brown the bimini and sweet corn thawed and well-drained, season with a little salt, and add the garlic rolled so that they also brown and add their flavor.

On the other hand, cook the chicken breasts on the grill or in a pan with extra virgin olive oil; you can add salt to taste or add a little Maldon salt after cooking.

Prepare the sauce to dress the dish; mix the soy sauce, the kimchi sauce, the sesame oil, the extra virgin olive oil, and the sesame seeds; if they are freshly toasted, the better. Serve time limit with the grilled corn, place the chicken breast on top, add a little flaked ñora, and season the chicken and vegetables with soy sauce, kimchi, and sesame.

Chicken Stuffed With Kale And Toum Sauce

Ingredients

- 4 small chicken breasts
- 6 ounces (160 grams) toum sauce (see recipe)
- 5 ounces (100-150 grams) of kale sprouts (small and tender leaves of this kale)
- one slice of fresh ginger
- 12 ounces (350 grams) of cocktail tomatoes
- freshly ground black pepper
- 1 tbsp. extra virgin olive oil
- 1 Pinch of salt
- 1 tsp of Anguilla (optional)
- a few flakes of Maldon salt.

STEPS

Clean the chicken breasts by trimming the 'sirloin' and, if necessary, part of them to remain in a portion. Open each chicken breast in halves like a book and season to taste.

Fill the chicken with the sauce (the amount can vary to taste), a little grated fresh ginger, and some kale sprouts. Tie the breasts with kitchen string to grill them later.

Brush the cast iron grill (or another type of grill, griddle, or pan) with extra virgin olive oil and cook the stuffed chicken breasts over medium-high heat, partially covering with a lid to make it easier for the thicker parts to take less time. in cooking. Flip it over when browned on one side and cook on the other. While the chicken is cooking, in another pan with a little extra virgin olive oil, sauté the rest of the kale with some neguilla seeds. You can also cook cocktail tomatoes in the pan or grill with the chicken.

Remove the kitchen string from the stuffed chicken and place it in the center of the plate. On one side, place the sautéed kale; around it, arrange the cocktail tomatoes and dress with a thread of raw extra virgin olive oil. Finish by sprinkling some toasted black beans and a little Maldon salt.

Chicken With Lemon And Hot Spices

Ingredients

- 4 chicken breasts
- 1 large lemon
- ½ tsp smoked salt
- ½ tsp shichimi togarashi
- ½ tsp ginger powder
- ½ tsp garlic powder
- w/ black pepper
- 8 sprigs of fresh coriander
- 3 garlic cloves
- oregano (optional)
- extra virgin olive oil
- Salt
- assorted lettuce leaves

STEPS

Start by preparing the spices to rub or marinate the chicken meat, wash the lemon skin very well and dry it. Grate it and put it in a small bowl. Add the smoked salt, shichimi, ginger and garlic powder, and pepper to taste. Wash and dry the coriander leaves and chop to incorporate it; finally, add a tablespoon of lemon juice, mix well, and reserve.
Prepare the chicken breasts, cut them into three filets, and rub the mixture of spices and lemon peel on the inner faces. Return the filets to form the breast again and tie it with kitchen string.
Heat a frying pan or grill with a little olive oil, put it over medium heat, place the flanged chicken breasts, season to taste, let them brown on one side, and then turn it over, seasoning again that they gild for the other. Due to the thickness of the pieces, it will take longer for the heat to reach the center, so cover the pan for about three to four minutes.

If necessary, add a little more olive oil. A couple of minutes before removing the chicken from the pan, add the previously peeled and sliced garlic to brown and add flavor. Finally, bathe each breast with approximately a tablespoon of natural lemon juice.
Arrange a bed of salad lightly dressed with extra virgin olive oil. Remove the kitchen string from the chicken breasts, and place them on the salad. Finish by grating a little more lemon zest over the chicken, adding the oregano, and letting any juices drip from the pan.

Chicken Breast With Boletus And Spinach

Ingredients

- 4 small chicken breasts
- 2-3 cloves of garlic
- 12 ounces (350 grams) of frozen boletus
- 3 ½ ounces (100 grams) of chicken broth
- 7 ounces (200 grams) of fresh spinach
- three sprigs of rosemary
- freshly ground black pepper

- a pinch of salt
- 1 tbsp. extra virgin olive oil
- 1 ½ ounces (30-40 grams) of Parmesan cheese (optional).

STEPS

Clean the breasts of any fat they may have and dry them with kitchen paper. Heat a large saucepan or frying pan with extra virgin olive oil. Season the chicken to taste; add the rosemary, and brown it over high heat.

Add the peeled and finely chopped garlic to the pan, adding a little more extra virgin olive oil beforehand if necessary. Give the garlic a couple of turns; with the high heat, they will immediately take on some color, and you have to prevent them from burning, so immediately pour the frozen boletus and the hot chicken broth once they are golden. Also add the spinach; at first, they will have a lot of volume, but with the help of a couple of spatulas, one in each hand, bring them closer to the bottom of the pan, placing them under the chicken so that they lose their volume with the heat. Season lightly and cook, without lowering the temperature of the fire, until the meat is done.

We cook over high heat at all times because both frozen boletus and fresh spinach need very little cooking; the former will not take long to defrost because they are poured with the hot broth, and the pan is over high heat. It is also interesting that the cooking is not very long so that the chicken is not dry inside, because when it is first marked on the outside to brown it, it is already partially cooked.

If the breasts are very thick, you can lower the heat so that the cooking is long and time to cook inside.

Serve the chicken breast accompanied by its garnish of boletus edulis and spinach and the juice in the pan. Finish with a dash of pepper and a few shavings of Parmesan cheese.

Chicken Skewers With Satay Sauce

Ingredients

- 4 chicken breasts
- 1 tsp ground coriander
- 1 tsp turmeric
- 1 tsp grated garlic
- freshly ground black pepper
- Salt
- extra virgin olive oil.

For the satay sauce
- 6-8 sprigs of fresh coriander
- 1 red chili
- 1 clove garlic
- three heaping tbsp peanut butter
- 2cm ginger root
- three tablespoons of kecap manis (or soy sauce and a pinch of sugar)
- 1 tsp of brown sugar
- 1 lemon
- 1 teaspoon of water (to lighten the sauce)
- a pinch of salt
- extra virgin olive oil or sesame oil (optional).

STEPS

As we have mentioned, we looked at Jamie Oliver's recipe, and he showed a trick to assemble the skewers; it is about threading the skewer sticks on the whole breasts, placing the four well together, interspersing the thick and thin parts. We wanted to do the test,t, but cutting the breasts lengthwise to similar-sized portions is not entirely possible, but it seemed like an interesting trick to quickly make the skewers. In the image gallery, you can get an idea of how we prepare them.

Once the skewers are threaded, the meat is cut to separate them. To tenderize the meat and make it more uneven, it is briefly pounded with the non-cutting part of the knife blade, another Jamie Oliver trick for a more crispy surface after cooking the chicken.

Once the chicken skewers are prepared, season them with the spices, rub them with a little extra virgin olive oil, and put them on the grill or a large frying pan over medium-high heat, depending on how thick the pieces are.

Meanwhile, prepare the sauce; it is as simple as putting all the ingredients in the processor or the blender glass and blending. Place the coriander leaves, the seeded chili pepper, the previously peeled garlic without the germ inside, the peanut butter, the minced ginger, the kecap manis sauce, the sugar, the grated lemon peel, and the lemon juice. Crush and taste to add water to obtain the desired texture and rectify salt.

Serve the freshly made chicken skewers accompanied by a small bowl of satay sauce. Add a trickle of oil to the sauce or skewers if you wish.

Aubergine Flatbread With Roasted Garlic And Sepionets

Ingredients

- four individual servings of coca bread (baguettes or flautas can be used)
- 3-4 sepionets
- one eggplant
- 1 small head of garlic
- parsley
- lumpfish roe
- extra virgin olive oil
- Salt.

STEPS

You can take advantage of the fact that you turn on the oven to make the coca bread, this time, we have made it with a dough of flour and beer, as you can see in the above link for breadsticks; you can also make this other recipe. When the coca is baked (if you decide to make it instead of using bread), roast the whole aubergine at 170-180° C until tender, about 30-40 minutes.

Next to the aubergine, roast the head of garlic from which you will have previously removed the crown and seasoned with olive oil and salt. Wrap it in aluminum foil to roast it. Check, after 20 minutes, if the garlic is tender, depending on its size, it will take more or less time; in the photograph in the image gallery, you can see what it should look like.

Meanwhile, put a saucepan on the heat with water and salt, cook the sepionets until they are tender, drain them, cut them into julienne strips, put them in a bowl, and add the chopped parsley, a drizzle of olive oil, and salt if necessary.

When the aubergine has cooled down a bit, and you can handle it, peel it and cut it into long strips. Peel the roasted garlic cloves and mash them with a fork until you get a garlic paste.

Spread the coca with the garlic paste, cover with the aubergine and add a pinch of salt. Then distribute the cuttlefish julienne and finally the lumpfish roe. Serve right away

Cuttlefish With Ginger And Coconut Milk

Ingredients (4-6 people)

- 21 ounces (600 grams) of clean cuttlefish
- one piece of ginger root (a nut)
- three garlic cloves
- 2 tablespoons of extra virgin olive oil
- one heaping tsp Gochu Jang (or red curry paste)
- 3 ½ ounces (100 grams) of coconut milk
- 2 tbsp. (20 grams) of soy sauce
- a pinch of salt
- 1 tablespoon of natural lemon juice
- six sprigs of fresh coriander
- ½ red onion
- 1 teaspoon sesame oil.

STEPS

Wash the cuttlefish and dry it well; cut it into bite-size pieces. Peel the ginger root and grate it. Peel the garlic cloves and grate them too, or if you prefer, use the garlic and ginger paste you have prepared.
Heat a frying pan with the extra virgin olive oil and fry the ginger and garlic paste over moderate heat. Add the cuttlefish and turn up the heat when it has done a little. Then add the Gochu Jang, give it a few turns. Add the coconut milk, soy sauce, a pinch of salt if necessary, and lemon juice; add the leaves of two chopped coriander sprigs. Cook over high heat, but not to the maximum, until the sauce reduces.
Peel and julienne the red onion and clean the remaining coriander leaves.
Serve the cuttlefish in casseroles or bowls and top with the onion and fresh coriander. Finish with a thread of sesame oil.

Asparagus Skewer And Cuttlefish Carpaccio With Parmesan

Ingredients

- one bunch of wild asparagus
- four toasts
- ¼ cuttlefish (unit)
- Parmesan
- extra virgin olive oil
- liquid smoke or Maldon smoked salt
- shichimi
- chive
- Salt.

STEPS

The cuttlefish must be frozen to cut it very thin, like a carpaccio. Clean the asparagus and chop them. Cut a few slices of Parmesan cheese with the peeler and arrange the toast on serving plates.
Once this is prepared, start by frying the asparagus in a pan with a little olive oil and salt to taste. Leave them slightly crispy and before removing them from the heat, add a few drops of liquid smoke or smoked salt (then control the regular salt you add). While you are putting the asparagus on the toast lightly watered with the juice that the asparagus has given off, put the cuttlefish in the pan with a little olive oil and salt, leave it for a few moments, just so that it takes temperature and is not completely raw. Place the cuttlefish carpaccio on the asparagus and the Parmesan cheese, the chives, sprinkle a little shichimi (optional), and a thread of extra virgin olive oil.

Cuttlefish Skewers With Romesco Sauce

Ingredients

For the skewers
- 12 small cuttlefish
- extra virgin olive oil
- fine sea salt
- red salt

For the romesco sauce
- 2 large plum tomatoes
- ½ head of garlic
- 1 ounces (30 grams) of peeled toasted almonds
- 1 ounces (30 grams) of peeled roasted hazelnut
- one slice of bread from the day before
- vinegar
- extra virgin olive oil
- Salt.

For the potatoes and avocado sauce
- 2 large potatoes
- 1 avocado
- 1 small spring onion
- 1 tsp zhug sauce (or other hot sauce)
- ten coriander leaves
- juice of half a lime
- extra virgin olive oil
- Maldon salt
- Salt.

STEPS

Prepare the romesco sauce so that it has time to cool down; you can make more quantity and thus have it to season the different dishes that are enriched with this sauce. To prepare it, you can follow the instructions in the Romesco Sauce post.

Prepare the skewers, for which you only have to clean the cuttlefish and thread them on a skewer stick, whether it is made of wood or stainless steel. When making the skewers (they should be served freshly made), put a little olive oil on a grill and cook them over medium-high heat, with a little salt, turning them from time to time so that they cook evenly until tender and slightly golden.

The potatoes can be presented in cylinders, as we have done and for which we have used a pasta cutter, or cut them into cubes (in either case, save the potato cuts to make a Parmentier). Put plenty of olive oil in a pan to fry them. As they have a significant thickness, it is convenient to confit them beforehand, and when they are tender, theory over high heat to take on a golden color.

While the potatoes are frying, prepare the avocado sauce, peel the fruit and put it in the blender glass with the lime juice, add the peeled and chopped onion, the zhug sauce, the coriander, salt, olive oil, and if necessary, you want, a little pepper. Blend until you get a thick avocado cream.

Serve three tablespoons of avocado sauce on the plates and place a cylinder of candied potato with a little Maldon salt and a coriander leaf on each of them. Paint the plate with a generous spoonful of romesco sauce and place the cuttlefish skewer seasoned with a pinch of red salt on it. Finish with a trickle of olive oil on the skewer and add, if you wish, some chopped dehydrated black olives.

Sautéed Chickpeas With Cuttlefish

Ingredients

- 21 ounces (600 grams) of cooked chickpeas
- 17 ounces (400-500 grams) of clean cuttlefish
- 4 cloves of garlic
- 1 slice of fresh ginger (optional)
- ½ lemon
- a pinch of Soso pink salt (salt with hibiscus, onion, two peppers, and smoked paprika)
- extra virgin olive oil
- fresh coriander
- fresh lemon verbena.

STEPS

The chickpeas should be cooked in advance, as you normally do, but without adding the ingredients of a stew. You can also buy some good canned or bulk cooked peas from a reputable market.

Wash and dry the cuttlefish well and cut it into cubes slightly larger than the chickpeas, put it in a colander, or dry it well before sautéing it. Peel the garlic cloves and cut them into slices. If you also want to add ginger, which will add aroma, flavor, and freshness to the dish, peel and grate it. Also, grate the skin of the lemon and reserve.

Heat a large frying pan with a couple of tablespoons of extra virgin olive oil, sauté the cuttlefish cubes for a few minutes, check that they are tender. Add salt and remove from heat.

In another larger frying pan, put a splash of extra virgin olive oil and add the well-drained chickpeas, sauté them over high heat, seasoning them with the pink salt, add the minced garlic and sauté for a few more minutes so that they brown and add flavor to the legume

Also incorporate the reserved cuttlefish and add a little hot paprika, give it a couple of turns and remove.

Serve the sautéed chickpeas with cuttlefish on plates and spread out the grated lemon peel, some fresh coriander and lemon verbena leaves, and a little more paprika. Finish with a thin stream of extra virgin olive oil and serve immediately.

Cuttlefish Casserole With Mushrooms

Ingredients

- 24 ounces (700 grams) of clean cuttlefish
- 12 ounces (350 grams) of shiitake mushrooms (or assorted mushrooms to taste)
- 8-10 young garlic cloves
- the green part of a spring onion
- 1 tsp fresh thyme
- ½ tsp freshly ground black pepper
- 2 tbsp oyster sauce
- A pinch of salt
- 1 teaspoon extra virgin olive oil.

STEPS

Wash the cuttlefish well, dry it and cut it into bite-size (small) pieces. Clean the mushrooms well and cut them into quarters or smaller, depending on size and taste. Peel the garlic cloves and cut them on the base, not very finely.

Remove the outer leaves from the green part of the onion and finely chop the inside. Strip the fresh thyme to add it to the stew.

Heat a saucepan with extra virgin olive oil, first sauté the spring garlic, let it brown over medium-high heat, then remove it if you want to serve it slightly crispy, if you prefer it to be well cooked, leave it in the casserole. In the oil in which the spring garlic has been made, add the mushrooms and cuttlefish, cook over medium heat, stirring from time to time, season with the green onion, thyme, black pepper, and salt to taste.

Mix well and let both cuttlefish and mushrooms expel their water, and then reduce it. At that time, add the oyster sauce and fry for a couple more minutes, stirring from time to time. Taste in case it is necessary to rectify the salt. Return the spring garlic to the pan, mix and remove from the heat.

Serve the cuttlefish stew with mushrooms on plates or in small saucepans, fresh from the heat. Warn your guests that they are going to suck their fingers.

Cuttlefish With Pickled Courgette

Ingredients

- 4 small cuttlefish
- 1 clove garlic
- 1 pickled zucchini (cut into sticks)
- 12 cherry tomatoes
- 1 purple onion
- 1 teaspoon of fresh coriander
- 1 teaspoon of shichimi togarashi
- a pinch of salt
- 1 teaspoonwith extra virgin olive oil.

STEPS

Prepare the vegetables first, drain the zucchini from the governing liquid, wash and dry the cherry tomatoes; in this case, we have used the pear-type ones because they usually come out a little sweeter, but you can choose the ones you like the most.

Peel the onion and cut it finely; if it is very itchy, you can soak it in cold water to soften it. Wash the coriander and dry it well before removing the leaves from the branches. Peel the garlic clove and cut it into slices.

Put a large skillet, or a frying pan, to heat with a little extra virgin olive oil to make the cuttlefish. These must be very clean and dry. When the grill is hot, add the cuttlefish, it is not convenient that the grill runs out of room, that the temperature is reduced, and that instead of being grilled, they are cooked, so if necessary, do them twice.

Make the cuttlefish by lightly browning them on both sides, adding salt to taste and the garlic to give it a little flavor. When they are done, remove them from the heat and proceed to serve.

Serve the cuttlefish on the plate and spread the pickled courgettes, the tomatoes, and the red onion, finishing with the fresh coriander, a little shichimi togarashi, and a trickle of extra virgin olive oil. Serve immediately

Cuttlefish Tagine With Lemon

Ingredients

- 4 small cuttlefish
- 1 onion
- ½ red bell pepper
- 1 clove garlic
- 2 small bay leaves or one large
- 1 lemon
- 6-8 stalks of fresh coriander
- 10-12 grains of coriander
- 10-12 black peppercorns
- a pinch of chili

- ½ tsp ground ginger
- ½ tsp smoked salt
- plain salt
- extra virgin olive oil.

STEPS

Put the base of the tajine on the fire with a little olive oil, add the onion and the pepper cut into brunoise, the clove of garlic with a blow and salt. Poach over low heat until these ingredients are very tender. Meanwhile, clean the cuttlefish well, wash the lemon, cut it into slices, and crush and mix the coriander grains, pepper, chili, ginger, and smoked salt in a mortar or Suribachi.

When the pepper and onion are soft, add the cuttlefish, a pinch of salt, and half of the spices from the mortar, in addition to the bay leaf, mix them with the sofrito and place a slice of lemon on each cuttlefish, seasoning them with the rest of the spices. Chop half of the fresh coriander and add it too. Cover the tagine and let it cook over medium heat. After ten minutes, turn the cuttlefish over and cover again, leaving another ten minutes. Depending on the size of the cuttlefish, this time will be enough for the meat to be very tender. If you are going to remove from the heat, there is still a lot of juice, let it cook over a higher heat and, without the lid for a couple of minutes, put the top of the cuttlefish down so that it browns slightly. Fry the remaining coriander leaves in hot oil until they are crispy; place them on absorbent kitchen paper when removing them.

Serve a couple of tablespoons of the onion and pepper sauce on the plates, place the cuttlefish and lemon wedge in the center, accompany the crispy cilantro and serve immediately.

Italian Chicken

Ingredients:

- 1 carrot, chopped
- ½ lb. / 680g. mushrooms
- 8 chicken thighs
- 1 cup tomato sauce
- 3 cloves garlic, crushed

STEPS

Season the chicken with salt and pepper.
Cover and marinate for 30 minutes.
Press the sauté setting in the Instant Pot.
Add 1 tablespoon of ghee.
Cook the carrots and mushrooms until soft.
Add the tomato sauce and garlic.
Add the chicken, tomatoes and olives.
Cook and mix well.
Seal the pot.
Set it to manual.
Cook at high pressure for 10 minutes.
Release the pressure naturally.

Turkey Verde with Brown Rice

Ingredients

- 2/3 cup chicken broth
- 1 ¼ cup brown rice
- 1 ½ lb./680g. turkey tenderloins
- 1 onion, sliced
- ½ cup salsa Verde

STEPS

Add the chicken broth and rice to the Instant Pot.
Top with the turkey, onion and salsa.
Cover the pot.
Set it to manual.
Cook at high pressure for 18 minutes.
Release the pressure naturally.
Wait for 8 minutes before opening the pot.

Turkey Meatloaf

Ingredients:

- ½ cup bread crumbs
- ¼ cup onion, chopped
- 1 lb.(450 g) lean ground turkey
- ¼ cup sun dried tomatoes, diced
- ½ cup feta cheese, crumbled

STEPS

Mix all the ingredients in a bowl.
Form a loaf and cover with foil.
Pour 1 cup of water into the Instant Pot.
Add the steamer basket inside.
Place the wrapped turkey mixture on top of basket.
Cover the pot.
Set it to manual.
Cook at high pressure for 35 minutes.

Turkey Lasagna

Ingredients:

- 4 tortillas
- 1 ¼ cup salsa
- ½ can refried beans
- 1 ½ cups cooked turkey
- 1 ¼ cup cheddar cheese, shredded

STEPS

Spray a small pan with oil.
Spread the refried beans on each tortilla.
Place the first tortilla inside the pan.
Add layers of the turkey, salsa and cheese.
Place another tortilla and repeat the layers.
Pour 1 cup of water inside the Instant Pot.
Place the layers on top of a steamer basket.
Place the basket inside the Instant Pot.
Choose manual setting.
Cook at high pressure for 10 minutes.

Eggplant Salad

Ingredients

- 1 large eggplant, washed and cubed
- 1 tomato, seeded and chopped
- 1 small onion, diced
- 2 tablespoons extra virgin olive oil
- ½ cup feta cheese, crumbled

STEPS

Pre-heat your outdoor grill to medium-high
Pierce the eggplant a few times using a knife/fork.
Cook the eggplants on your grill for about 15 minutes until they are charred.

Keep it on the side and allow them to cool.
Remove the skin from the eggplant and dice the pulp.
Transfer the pulp to mixing bowl and add onion, tomato, olive oil, feta cheese.
Mix well and chill for 1 hour.
Season with salt and enjoy!

Tender Watermelon and Radish Salad

Ingredients

- 10 medium beets, peeled and cut into 1-inch chunks
- 1 teaspoon extra virgin olive oil
- 4 cups seedless watermelon, diced
- 1 tablespoon fresh thyme, chopped
- 1 lemon, juiced

STEPS

Pre-heat your oven to 350 degrees Fahrenheit
Take a small bowl and add beets, olive oil and toss well to coat the beets.
Roast beets for 25 minutes until tender
Transfer to large bowl and cool them.
Add watermelon, kale, radishes, thyme, lemon juice, and toss.
Season sea salt and pepper.

Tasty Yogurt and Cucumber Salad

Ingredients

- 5-6 small cucumbers, peeled and diced
- 1 (8 ounces) container plain Greek yogurt
- 2 garlic cloves, minced
- 1 tablespoon fresh mint, minced
- Sea salt and fresh black pepper

STEPS

Take a large bowl and add cucumbers, garlic, yogurt, mint.
Season with salt and pepper.
Refrigerate the salad for 1 hour and serve.

Herbed Up Feisty Baby Potatoes

Ingredients

- 2 pounds (900 g) new yellow potatoes, scrubbed and cut into wedges
- 2 tablespoons extra virgin olive oil
- 2 teaspoons fresh rosemary, chopped
- 1 teaspoon garlic powder
- $\frac{1}{2}$ teaspoon freshly ground black pepper and salt

STEPS

Pre-heat your oven to 400 degrees Fahrenheit.
Line baking sheet with aluminum foil and set it aside.
Take a large bowl and add potatoes, olive oil, garlic, rosemary, sea salt and pepper.
Spread potatoes in single layer on baking. sheet and bake for 35 minutes.
Serve and enjoy!

Mesmerizing Brussels and Pistachios

Ingredients

- 1 pound (450g) Brussels sprouts, tough bottom trimmed and halved lengthwise
- 1 tablespoon extra-virgin olive oil
- Salt and pepper as needed

- ½ cup roasted pistachios, chopped
- Juice of ½ lemon

STEPS

Pre-heat your oven to 400 degrees Fahrenheit.
Line a baking sheet with aluminum foil and keep it on the side.
Take a large bowl and add Brussels sprouts with olive oil and coat well.
Season sea salt, pepper, spread veggies evenly on sheet.
Bake for 15 minutes until lightly caramelized.
Remove oven and transfer to a serving bowl.
Toss with pistachios and lemon juice.
Serve warm and enjoy!

Fancy Greek Orzo Salad

Ingredients

- 1 cup orzo pasta, uncooked
- ½ cup fresh parsley, minced
- 6 teaspoons olive oil
- 1 onion, chopped
- 1 ½ teaspoons oregano

STEPS

Cook your orzo and drain them.
Add to a serving dish.
Add 2 teaspoons of oil.
Take another dish and add parsley, onion, remaining oil and oregano.
Season with salt, pepper according to your flavor.
Pour the mixture over orzo and let it chill for 24 hours.
Serve and enjoy at lunch!

Cheesy Roasted Broccoli

Ingredients

- 2 head broccoli, cut into florets
- 2 tablespoon extra-virgin olive oil + lemon juice
- 2 teaspoon garlic, minced
- a pinch of salt
- ½ cup parmesan cheese, grated

STEPS

Pre-heat your oven to 400 degrees F.
Lightly grease the baking sheet with olive oil and keep it on the side.
Take a large bowl and add broccoli with 2 tablespoons olive oil, garlic, lemon juice, and salt.
Spread mix on the baking sheet in single layer and sprinkle parmesan cheese.
Bake for 10 minutes until tender.
Transfer broccoli to serving the dish.

Mediterranean Kale Dish

Ingredients

- 12 cups kale, chopped
- 2 tablespoons lemon juice
- 1 tablespoon olive oil
- 1 teaspoon soy sauce
- Salt and pepper as needed

STEPS

Add a steamer insert to your Saucepan.
Fill the saucepan with water up to the bottom of the steamer.
Cover and bring water to boil (medium-high heat).

Add kale to the insert and steam for 7-8 minutes.
Take a large bowl and add lemon juice, olive oil, salt, soy sauce, and pepper.
Mix well and add the steamed kale to the bowl.
Toss and serve.
Enjoy!

Shrimp in White Wine

Ingredients:
- 1 tablespoon butter
- 1 tablespoon garlic, minced
- 2 lb. (shrimp, peeled and deveined
- 1/2 cup chicken stock
- 1/2 cup white wine

STEPS

Set the Instant Pot to sauté. Add the butter and the garlic, cook for 30 seconds.
Pour in the stock and wine to deglaze.
Add the shrimp. Season with salt and pepper.
Cover the pot. Set it to manual and cook at high pressure for 1 minute.
Release the pressure naturally.

CHAPTER 7

Dinner

Recipes

Pumpkin Cream Recipe With Trumpet Of Death, Cheese Crumbs, And Confit Garlic Cream

Ingredients

- 9 ounces (250 grams) of trumpets of death
- 1 clove garlic
- one sprig of curly parsley
- 25 ounces (700 grams) of roasted pumpkin
- ½ roasted red onion
- 17 ounces (500 grams) of ham broth or other to taste
- ½ tsp ginger powder
- ½ tsp grated nutmeg
- ½ tsp freshly ground black pepper
- 1 tsp sweet and sour Vera paprika
- A Pinch of salt
- 1 tablespoon of extra virgin olive oil
- 4 tablespoons of cured Idiazabal cheese
- 4 tablespoons of confit garlic cream with soy and honey

STEPS

Clean the trumpets of death, try not to get them wet, cut the base that may have soil, and remove any leaves or brush attached. Peel the garlic clove and finely chop it. Heat a frying pan with a little extra virgin olive oil. When hot, add the mushrooms, parsley, and minced garlic and sauté until tender, a few minutes. Add salt and remove from heat. The pumpkin must be roasted in advance; it can be freshly made. We like it more roasted in the oven than cooked or boiled, but you can make this cream with pumpkin made to your liking. When we roast the squash in the oven, we usually also roast a few heads of garlic and onions for other recipes.

Put the roasted pumpkin in the food processor and add the roasted onion, broth, spices, ginger, nutmeg, black pepper, and paprika. Also, add salt to taste, keeping in mind that the pumpkin is sweet and how salty the added broth is; better to stay short; you can always add more salt at the end. Blend everything until you get a homogeneous cream, then, without stopping beating, add a splash of extra virgin olive oil to bind the cream further. Taste it and rectify salt or spices if necessary. Before serving, put it in a saucepan, bring it to a boil and turn off the heat. Heat the black trumpets if they have cooled.

Serve the roasted butternut squash soup in bowls and dish out the sautéed trumpets of death. Then coarsely grate the cheese and distribute it too. Serve a spoonful of confit garlic cream with soy and honey, which gives it a point of delicious flavor, and to give it a touch of color, sprinkle a pinch of chopped ñora.

Pumpkin And Clove Cream With Kale Sprouts

Ingredients

- 9 ounces (250 grams) of white leek
- 5 ounces (150 grams) of parsnip
- 32 ounces (850-900 grams) butternut squash without skin
- 3 cloves
- a thick slice of fresh ginger
- ½ tsp allspice
- 25 ounces (700 grams) of vegetable broth
- 1 tsp anchovy brine (optional)
- A Pinch of salt
- 1 tablespoon extra virgin olive oil
- 1 tsp peeled hemp seeds
- four handfuls of kale sprouts.

STEPS

Peel the leeks, reserve the green part for ano, the recipe, and cut the white part first and then into slices. Peel the parsnip and do the same; cut it into not very thick half-moons. Peel the pumpkin; if it seems too hard, you can use this trick to make the skin softer and easier to peel. Next, cut the pulp into small cubes, they do not have to be the same, but they do have to be of a similar size.

Heat a saucepan with a good splash of extra virgin olive oil, add the leek, parsnip, and pumpkin, add salt to taste and the cloves, mix well. Grate the fresh ginger and add it to the pot together with the freshly ground allspice, and fry for a few minutes until the vegetables begin to color.

Pour the broth into the pot, turn up the heat and let it come to a boil. At that time, lower the heat and cook until the pumpkin is very tender. Then, remove from the heat and add the anchovy brine or a splash of tamari or soy sauce; the cream will gain intensity in flavor.

Crush the vegetables until you get a fine cream, taste, rectify salt or spices, and bring to a boil again. Remove from heat and reserve.

Wash the kale sprouts well (if you can't find this sprout, you can try another one that you like, but not as fine as alfalfa, for example, so that you can notice the crunchy texture and freshness when chewing)), which will add a fresh and crunchy touch to the cream, and drain well.

Serve the pumpkin and clove cream in deep plates or bowls; add some peeled hemp seeds, providing a fresh and dried fruit note around the kale sprouts that you will have put in the center. Finish with a trickle of extra virgin olive oil.

Roasted Pumpkin Cream With Sage

Ingredients

- ½ pumpkin (we will need 14 ounces/400 grams of roasted pumpkin to make the cream)
- 3 sprigs of fresh sage
- 1 teaspoon of garlic powder
- ½ tsp allspice
- a pinch of black pepper
- 5 ounces (150 grams) of broth (it can be meat, poultry, or vegetables, each one will provide its strongest or mildest flavor)
- 3 ½ ounces (100 grams) of milk (you can put cream to cook or half and a half to make it creamier)
- 1 tsp sweet and sour smoked paprika
- croutons
- chive
- fresh coriander
- Salt
- extra virgin olive oil.

STEPS

Prepare the pumpkin to roast it in the oven; you can do it without peeling it as we explained in the post Cooking tricks: Peel and cut a pumpkin, first bake the pumpkin very clean, whole, so that the skin softens, and then cut it into segments and remove the skin with ease.

Put the pumpkin slices or wedges seasoned with extra virgin olive oil, sage, allspice, black pepper, salt, and garlic powder on an oven tray, although this can replace this with whole garlic cloves like this, and the taste is much better. Still, when making the pumpkin cream on this occasion, we had run out of stock.

Bake the pumpkin at 180º C for 40-60 minutes, until tender and slightly toasted. Then transfer it to the blender glass and add the broth, milk or cream, paprika, and extra virgin olive oil. Blend until you get a fine cream and try to see if it is necessary to rectify the salt.

Prepare the croutons or croutons and chop the chives and coriander.

Serve the roasted pumpkin cream with sage in bowls or deep plates, present the croutons in the center, distribute the chives and coriander, and finish with a trickle of extra virgin olive oil.

Pumpkin Cream With Roasted Chickpeas And Avocado

Ingredients

- 35 ounces (1 kilo) pumpkin (without skin or seeds)
- 20 ounces (600 ml) of water or vegetable broth
- a pinch of salt
- 2 cloves of garlic
- 1 slice of fresh ginger
- ½ sweet onion
- 1 tsp of smoked paprika from La Vera
- ½ tsp xanthan (optional)
- 1 tsp of zaatar with green mango and ñora (see recipe)
- ¼ red radicchio
- 10 ½ ounces (300 grams) of cooked chickpeas
- ¾ avocado
- 1 tablespoon of extra virgin olive oil
- A pinch of salt.

STEPS

Cut the squash into regular pieces, not very thick, to cook faster. Please put it in a microwave-safe container and program for 8 minutes at maximum power. Meanwhile, heat the water or broth, peel the garlic cloves and slice them, peel the ginger and grate it, peel the onion and chop it brunoise.

Heat a frying pan with a splash of extra virgin olive oil and sauté the garlic, onion, and ginger; when they have taken on a little color, remove the pan from the heat, add the smoked paprika, mix, and reserve.

When the pumpkin is cooked, put it in the blender jar and add the water or broth, the fried garlic, ginger, onion, paprika, xanthan, and a drizzle of extra virgin olive oil.

The xanthan helps to emulsify the cream; if you don't use it, you can add extra virgin olive oil or a little cream with high-fat content; it also helps to emulsify. Still, it will be necessary to rectify the seasoning because it will soften the flavor of the cream. Cream, try to put it to the point, to your liking. Before serving the pumpkin cream, could you bring it to a boil?

Heat a frying pan with a little extra virgin olive oil and toast the cooked chickpeas with the red radicchio cut into julienne strips, keep moving so that they cook evenly, and when it is almost ready, add the zaatar, mix, and cook.

Serve the pumpkin cream with smoked paprika in deep dishes, distribute the chickpeas with the radicchio in the center and add the diced avocado. To finish, dress with a thread of extra virgin olive oil.

Pumpkin Cream With Light Escarole And Parmesan Stew

Ingredients (4-6 people)

- 35 ounces (1 kilo) roasted pumpkin
- 1 shallot
- 1 clove garlic
- 1 slice of fresh ginger
- 1 tablespoon of paprika
- $1/2$ tsp allspice
- 1 tsp tarragon
- 12 ounces (350 grams) of cream to cook
- 12 ounces (350 grams) of vegetable broth
- a pinch of salt
- 1 tablespoon extra virgin olive oil.

For the garnish
- 1 shallot
- $1/4$ endive
- 1 tablespoon of raisins
- 1 tablespoon of pine nuts
- $1/2$ tsp black sesame seeds
- 3 ounces (60-90 grams) of Parmesan cheese (in one piece)
- a pinch of smoked paprika
- 1 tsp sesame oil
- $1/2$ tsp extra virgin olive oil
- A pinch of salt.

STEPS

Roast the pumpkin in the oven in advance, although you can also make this cream with boiled or steamed pumpkin. Peel the shallot, garlic, and ginger grate the latter. Heat a pot with a little extra virgin olive oil and fry the shallot, garlic, and ginger.

When the shallot is very soft, add the chopped roasted pumpkin and season with paprika, allspice, and tarragon, give it a couple of turns so that it is impregnated with the flavors of the spices and that the heat enhances them, and add the liquid cream, the broth and the amount of salt that is necessary.

Bring to a boil and cook for one or two minutes, then remove from the heat and blend until you obtain a fine and homogeneous cream. The cream can be made as thin or thick as you like; you have to play with the amount of liquid you add. Taste to rectify if necessary, and bring to a boil again. Then remove from the fire.

Put a little extra virgin olive oil and sesame oil in a large frying pan, poach the chopped endive leaves, take advantage of the darkest endive leaves for this light stew, and reserve the lighter ones for a salad. Add the chopped shallot, raisins, pine nuts, and black sesame seeds to the escarole. When the leaves are tender, remove them from heat.

Serve the roasted pumpkin cream in deep dishes and place the light escarole stew in the center. Add a few slices of Parmesan cheese that you can make with a vegetable peeler, and sprinkle a little smoked paprika.

Pumpkin Cream, Ham And Pine Nuts

Ingredients (4-6 people)

- one leek
- one slice of fresh ginger
- 1 tablespoon extra virgin olive oil
- Salt
- 35 ounces (1 kilo) of pumpkin (weighed once roasted)
- 1 tsp chopped sage
- ½ tsp allspice
- nutmeg
- 17 ounces (500 grams) of chicken broth
- 8 ounces (240 grams) of evaporated milk
- eight slices of serrano ham
- eight chive leaves (optional)
- 2 tablespoons of pine nuts.

STEPS

As we indicate in the ingredients, the pumpkin's weight is once roasted; it is generally how we prepare it to make different recipes. You can roast the pumpkin in the oven or cook it in a pot, whichever you like best.

Peel the leek, wash it well, drain it, cut it in half, and finely chop it. Peel the ginger, the thickness of the slice can be somewhat thicker than a euro coin, but if you want to intensify its flavor, you can put a little more, with this amount, it is very soft, if you do not know the taste of all the guests, it is better to put it sparingly.

Heat a pot with a little extra virgin olive oil and poach the leek and ginger, peeled and finely chopped, over medium heat, add a little salt, and stir. When the leek is tender, add the chopped pumpkin, it should be soft after cooking, and a paste is made simply by flattening it a bit.

Season with the sage, allspice, nutmeg, and salt to taste, fry for a few minutes so that the pumpkin is impregnated with the aroma of the spices, and moisten with the broth (if you prefer, it can be made with vegetables). Bring to a boil.

Once it has started to boil, cook for a couple of minutes, remove the pot from the heat and blend, add the evaporated milk and blend again until you obtain a fine and homogeneous cream. Taste the cream if it is necessary to rectify salt or any spice. Return the pot to the heat and bring it back to a boil. Cook for a couple of minutes and turn off the heat.

Prepare the ham; form a cylinder with each slice; it is not necessary to tie it with chives to keep it. Put a frying pan to heat, and first toast the pine nuts over moderate heat and move them to be well toasted. Remove the pine nuts and raise the heat, place the slices of ham by the closing part, let it roast and turn it over until its entire contour is crispy.

Serve the pumpkin cream and place two cylinders of ham in the center; you can put the fresh and tasty chives and add a touch of color. Finish by distributing the pine nuts, a little sad, age, and a few extra virgin olive oil drops.

Pumpkin And Coconut Cream

Ingredients (4-6 people)
- 35 ounces / 1 kg. of peeled and chopped pumpkin
- 2 small or one large leek
- 1 tsp curry
- ½ tsp turmeric
- ½ tsp thyme
- black pepper to taste
- nutmeg
- 1 cup (300 milliliters) of coconut milk
- ½ cup (100 milliliters) of milk (or a little more to rectify the density of the cream)
- ten prawns
- grated coconut
- Salt
- . extra virgin olive oil.

STEPS

Pocha in a frying pan or large saucepan with a good jet of olive oil, the chopped pumpkin with the peeled and chopped leek, season with salt and pepper to taste, and let it cook over low heat until the pumpkin is tender about 20 minutes, also It will depend on the size to which you have chopped the pumpkin.

If you see that the casserole is very dry, add cow's milk in small doses to help cook the pumpkin. When it is already tender and begins to melt, add the coconut milk, curry, turmeric, thyme, nutmeg, and adjust salt and pepper. Continue cooking for ten more minutes.

Pour the result into the Thermomix glass or a large bowl and blend until you get a fine cream. If you want it to be lighter, add a little milk. Taste and rectify salt or spices if necessary.

Grill the prawns; you can do them with the shell and then peel them, or peel them first (reserving the head and the shell to make a sauce or broth) and give them a couple of turns in a pan, naturally with salt to taste. Serve the pumpkin and coconut cream in deep plates or bowls and place two or three peeled prawns in the center, sprinkle a little grated coconut, and finish with a trickle of olive oil. A sprig of dill or cilantro will add color to the dish.

Pumpkin Cream With Smoked Herring Roe And Black Garlic

Ingredients

- 14 ounces (400 grams) of roasted pumpkin
- 3 ½ ounces (100 grams) of cooked chickpeas
- 8 ounces (200-240 grams) of seafood broth
- one small garlic clove
- a pinch of salt
- 1 tablrespoon extra virgin olive oil
- 4 tsp smoked herring roe
- two cloves of black garlic.

STEPS

Once you have the roasted pumpkin (if you have never done it, you can never follow this recipe), put it in the blender jar. Add the chickpeas that you will have previously cooked, although you can also resort to the good preservation of this length ume for this type of elaboration.
The richer the seafood broth you make, the better this pumpkin cream will be; you can also do it with fish, for example, monkfish, galleys, prawns... Pour the hot broth, along with the chickpeas, also hot, into the blender glass with roasted pumpkin.
Add the peeled garlic and salt to taste, depending on how salty the broth is. Also, add a good splash of extra virgin olive oil and blend until you get a fine, homogeneous cream. You can make it as thick or light as you like, adding more or less seafood stock. Reserve the hot pumpkin cream until serving time. Peel the black garlic and cut them into slices to put three in each appetizer glass.

Pour the pumpkin and seafood cream into the appetizer cups, distribute the smoked herring roe and the black garlic in the center of each one. Finish with some edible flowers if you have them, for example, oregano, chives, and a trickle of extra virgin olive oil. Serve immediately, hot.

Pumpkin And Turnip Cream

Ingredients

- 18 ounces (500 grams) of pumpkin
- 10 ½ ounces (300 grams) of turnips
- 1 purple onion
- 2 cloves of garlic
- 13 ½ ounces (400 milliliters) of milk
- 1 tablespoon of hatch miso
- fresh ginger
- black pepper
- Sesame oil
- extra virgin olive oil
- Salt.

STEPS

Peel and dice the squash and turnips, heat a saucepan with a drizzle of olive oil, and fry both ingredients, seasoned to taste. Meanwhile, peel and chop the onion and garlic.
After about ten minutes, add the onion to the pan, stir from time to time and sauté over medium heat until the onion is poached, then add the garlic, and when it has browned, add the milk, miso, grated fresh ginger, and let cook for about 15-20 minutes. After this time, remove the pan from the heat and transfer the preparation to a bowl or to the glass of the Thermomix to blend. You will obtain a fine cream that you can

lighten if you wish with a little water or milk, but the texture must be optimal following these quantities.
Serve the pumpkin cream with turnips in small individual bowls, drizzle with a few drops of sesame oil and decorate with basil, chives, or a sprig of thyme.

Pumpkin Cream With Mi Cuit Foie And Black Truffle

Ingredients

- 25 ounces (700 grams) of peeled and seeded pumpkin
- 3 ½ ounces(100 grams)of leek
- 2 cups (½ liter) of water
- 1 ounces / 40 grams of cooking cream (milk cream)
- 1 tsp of ground spice mix (thyme, oregano, cardamom, cumin, chili, ginger, black pepper, allspice, coriander, mustard, nutmeg... you can add fewer spices to enhance certain aromas)
- 3 ½ ounces/100 grams of foie mi cuit
- 1 tablespoon/8-10 grams of fresh black truffle (Tuber melanosporum)
- 4 tsp freshly grated Parmesan (optional)
- extra virgin olive oil
- sugar (if you want to caramelize the foie)
- flake salt
- plain salt.

STEPS

Put a large-based pot or casserole over the heat with a little extra virgin olive oil once you have the pumpkin diced and the leek peeled and julienned. Reserve two or three pumpkin pieces the size of a cereal bar to mark it later in a pan and serve it cut into small cubes, offering another texture on the plate.
Lightly brown the chopped pumpkin and the leek, adding salt to taste, at a moderate temperature. When it begins to soften and take on color, add the spices and give it a few turns so that they take temperature and begin to release their flavor. Add the water and bring to a boil. When it starts to boil, lower the heat and cook until the pumpkin is very tender, the time will depend on its size, but it is easy to check that its texture is well done. Crush the pumpkin with the blender or in the Thermomix, and return it to the pan; add the cream and mix it well with the pumpkin cream, bring to a boil and then remove from the heat. Try it in case you need to rectify salt or spices. Booking.
Sear the pumpkin tacos, as we mentioned, in a non-stick pan with a little extra virgin olive oil. When they have taken color on both sides, remove the pumpkin from the pan and cut it into small cubes.

Cut the foie mi cut into four portions and place them on a surface where you can use the torch. Cover the surface with sugar and burn it with the kitchen torch. Finally, slice the black truffle.
Serve the Pumpkin cream by placing the foie mi-cut in the center, which you can raise on the plate by placing a cube of pumpkin underneath. Distribute the rest of the cubes on the plates and then distribute the laminated black truffle on the hottest surface of the plate so that its aroma and flavor emanate. However, you can always heat the whole in the preheated oven, being careful not to alter the texture of the foie. Add a few flakes of salt to the pumpkin cubes and finish with a few extra virgin olive oil drops to give the dish a shine and flavor. You can

always use truffle oil if you don't have a black truffle. For those who want it, serve a tablespoon of grated Parmesan cheese on the side of the plate or in a bowl at the table.

Chickpea And Pumpkin Hummus

Ingredients (4-6 people)

- 10 ½ ounces/300 grams of cooked chickpeas (and a little broth)
- 7 ounces /200 grams of roasted or cooked pumpkin
- 2 tablespoons of tahini
- 2 cloves of garlic
- a splash of natural lemon juice
- 1 ½ ounces (50 ml) of extra virgin olive oil
- 3-4 sprigs of coriander (or parsley)
- 1 tsp paprika from La Vera or paprika
- 1 tsp cumin powder
- freshly ground black pepper to taste
- a pinch of salt

STEPS

Drain the chickpeas, if you cook them yourself, to later add the necessary broth because depending on the humidity that the pumpkin retains, you will need more or less. Oven-roasted squash will contain less water than boiled or steamed squash.

In any case, you must make the pumpkin in advance and let it cool. You can also make hummus by buying cooked chickpeas, either canned or in bulk, at your market. It can be interesting to rinse the legume in the first case, especially for the taste.

Put the chickpeas and the chopped pumpkin in the glass of the blender or food processor. Add the toasted sesame tahini (there is also raw sesame), the peeled garlic cloves, the extra virgin olive oil, the coriander leaves, the Vera paprika, and the cumin. Also, season with freshly ground black pepper to taste and salt.

Crush all the ingredients and add a little broth or, failing that, water until you get a dense puree as fine or rustic as you want; everyone may like a texture for the hummus. Serve the pumpkin hummus on a deep plate or a bowl and add some cooked chickpeas, some coriander leaves, a little paprika, and to finish, add a dash of extra virgin olive oil. Accompany with a good freshly baked or freshly toasted flatbread, hot and crispy.

Pumpkin Gazpacho

Ingredients
- 14 ounces (400 grams) of pumpkin without skin or seeds
- 21 ounces (600 grams) of pear tomato
- 4 ounces (120 grams) of red pepper
- 3 ounces (80 grams) of cucumber (without skin)
- 1 ½ ounces (40 grams) of purple onion (or spring onion)
- one clove garlic
- 2 ounces (50 grams) of sitting bread
- 2 ounces (60 grams) of extra virgin olive oil
- pinch of salt
- four slices of Serrano ham (optional)
- one thin slice of pumpkin
- 1 teaspoon of garlic sprouts (Rock chives)
- extra virgin olive oil.

STEPS

The weight of the ingredients indicated is clean, without skin, seeds, stalk... Prepare them as you normally do, chop the pumpkin and remove the skin and seeds, wash the tomatoes and remove the stalk; if you make the gazpacho in a food processor Thermomix, no need to peel them. Wash and chop the red pepper, peel the cucumber, and cut it into pieces; peel the purple onion and chop it.

Finally, peel the garlic clove and put all the prepared ingredients in the Thermomix glass. Add the chopped bread, the extra virgin olive oil, the salt (bearing in mind that crispy ham will be added later, which is very salty), and, if you wish, a dash of vinegar.

Blend at progressive speed (3-5-7-9) for four or five minutes until you obtain a dense, fine, and homogeneous gazpacho. Test it and rectify it if necessary. Let it rest in the refrigerator to serve it very cold.

Prepare the garnish for the pumpkin gazpacho, put the ham spread out on a plate, on absorbent kitchen paper, and put it in the microwave, first for a minute, so that it dries out, if it is not crisp enough, put it a little more. Once cool, break it into small pieces with your hands.

Chop the thin slice of raw pumpkin into brunoise and prepare the sprouts of soft garlic; alternatively, you can use little chives that add color and a flavor found in gazpacho.

Serve the pumpkin gazpacho very fresh, distributing the diced pumpkin garnish, crispy ham, and garlic sprouts in the center. Accompany a few slices of village bread and enjoy.

Hake With Tomatoes Marinated In Soy

Ingredients

- 4 hake loins
- 10 ½ ounces /250-300 grams of assorted cherry tomatoes
- one clove garlic
- one thick slice of fresh ginger
- four sprigs of fresh coriander
- 1 tsp of sugar
- 1 tsp of soy sauce
- three tender garlic
- Soho pink salt (hibiscus, onion, two peppers, and smoked paprika)
- 1 tbsp extra virgin olive oil.

STEPS

The day before, prepare the tomatoes to marinate, wash them well, cut them in half, and put them in a bowl.

Peel the garlic and ginger, grate the two ingredients, and add them to the tomato container. Wash and dry half the cilantro and chop it to add it to the tomatoes, also add the sugar and soy sauce, add the necessary amount so that they are well impregnated but not swimming in soy sauce, cover the base of the dish and from time to time turn it over so that it continues to soak up the flavors of the marinade.

The tomatoes well covered, in a container with a lid or covered with transparent film, leave them overnight in the refrigerator. Remove them before making food.

Clean the hake loins of bones, dry them well, and reserve. Peel the garlic cloves and cut them into small pieces on the bias. Heat a large frying pan with a splash of extra virgin olive oil.

When it is hot, add the spring garlic, sauté them for a few minutes, until they are to your liking, you can leave them crispy or soft; in the first case, remove them from the pan before cooking the fish in the oil that has been flavored, in the second, leave them to cook them with the hake.

Cook fish skin side first, cook until crisp, then flip to cook the other side. Once the fish is done, please turn off the heat but keep the pan over it and add the marinated tomatoes with the soy sauce and the reserved chopped fresh coriander. In principle, it is about heating the tomatoes, not cooking them, although you can sauté them for a few minutes if you want them to be slightly cooked and soft.

Serve the hake and spread over it and on the sides, the sautéed cherry tomatoes with their sauce, the spring garlic and a thread of extra virgin olive oil add a little pink salt to the fish or to taste, remember that the soy sauce on the plate is already salty.

Baked Bream With Arugula And Ham

Ingredients
- four sea bream portion
- 1 lemon
- two leeks
- 1 tsp of salt
- 1 tbsp of extra virgin olive oil
- a pinch of thyme
- a pinch of freshly ground pepper
- 5 ounces/150 grams of txacolí
- 2 ½ ounces /125 grams of diced Serrano ham
- 2 ounces/50 grams of arugula
- a handful of sliced almonds.

STEPS

Clean the giltheads well; they must be whole, with the central spine and the head, but gutted and scaled. Turn on the oven, with heat up and down, to 200° C.
Wash the lemon well and cut it into slices. Peel the leeks, wash them well, and cut them half lengthwise and crosswise. Place the leeks in the oven, which will support the fish, after pouring a thread of extra virgin olive oil. Make some superficial cuts in the skin of the sea bream, place a slice of lemon inside, season to taste, add a little thyme, then place the fish on top of the leek halves. Pour the txacolí onto the tray and when the oven has reached temperature, place it in the oven for approximately 20-25 minutes. Depending on the size of the sea bream, the time may vary. When about five minutes of cooking are left, remove the tray from the oven and add the arugula, ham, and sliced almonds, but the golden ones back in the oven, and finish cooking, the skin will be slightly golden, the arugula will have lost its volume, the ham will have released its flavor, the almonds will be toasted...
Serve the sea bream on each plate, accompanied by the resulting juice with ham, almonds, arugula, and leek. Finish with a trickle of extra virgin olive oil and some fresh arugula leaves.

Grilled Sea Bream With Clams

Ingredients

- four sea bream portion
- 17 ounces /500 grams of fresh clams
- garlic cloves
- 2-3 a few leaves of fresh parsley
- a splash of white wine (optional)

- 1 tsp of ground chili (if you want spicy) or ground ñora
- 1 tbsp of extra virgin olive oil
- A pinch of salt.

STEPS

Clean the gilt heads and open them like a butterfly, removing the central spine and the head. You can order it at the fishmonger like this. Once clean, dry them with absorbent kitchen paper.

It is best to leave the clams in salted water beforehand to clean them well and ensure that they do not have any sand; normally, a couple of hours before cooking is recommended; you can read more about it here.

Peel the garlic cloves, cut them into slices, and finely chop the parsley. Another option is to use freeze-dried parsley, better than the usually dried parsley; it is a resource for when you cannot have fresh parsley.

To cook the clams, heat a frying pan with a splash of extra virgin olive oil and add the bivalves. Add a little wine and a pinch of salt, and chopped parsley if you wish. Cover the pan and cook until all the clams are open, remove from heat, and reserve.

To make the sea breams, heat the grill with a little extra virgin olive oil; when it is hot, add the fish on the skin side and cook it until it is toasted. Add the chopped parsley and the minced garlic to brown and flavor the fish. On the skin side, it should be cooked longer than on the other side; in this way, a juicier fish is obtained, although you like to mark it so that it is also golden on the surface. So once it's done on the skin side, flip it over and keep the brown just long enough for it to take on a bit of color.

Serve the grilled sea bream with its garlic and accompany it with some clams, seasoning the fish lightly with a little of its juice. Take him to the table right away and eat.

Low-Temperature Teriyaki Cod

Ingredients

- four cod filets to the point of salt
- 8 ounces /250 grams of round green beans
- 1 tsp of eriyaki sauce
- 1 tablespoon of sesame seeds
- 8 tender garlic
- one tip of Riojan joy (hot peppers)
- extra virgin olive oil
- Salt.

STEPS

Prepare the cod (desalted and to the point of salt), cut the loins so that there is a thick block (you can reserve the cuts, for example, to make a cod brandade). Brush them with teriyaki sauce and wrap them in plastic wrap, sealing them well. Reserve in the refrigerator. You can do this step a couple of hours before you start cooking.

Prepare the green beans, trim them and wash them well. Put a saucepan with plenty of water and a little salt and cook them for about five minutes, so they are crispy or longer if you prefer them more tender. Cool them in ice water and dress them with a little extra virgin olive oil when they are done. Booking.

Put a pot with water (enough to submerge the fish) to heat over medium heat; you will need a thermometer to know when it reaches 149°F/ 60-65° C; at that moment, introduce the cod packages.

Keeping the temperature at around 149°F/ 60° C, cook the cod for approximately ten minutes. Then remove it from the water and peel it off the cling film.

While the cod is cooking, put a little extra virgin olive oil in a frying pan, peel and chop the spring garlic and the piece of Riojan joy. Sauté green beans, garlic, bell pepper, and sesame seeds over medium-high heat.

Serve a bed of green beans, dressing if you wish, with a little teriyaki sauce and a few drops of extra virgin olive oil. Place the cod loin on the beans. Paint again with teriyaki sauce and finish with a fine thread of extra virgin olive oil.

Salmon With Broccoli And Almond Cream

Ingredients

- four servings of fresh salmon (about 5 ounces/150 grams each)
- 4 ounces/110 grams of leek
- 5 ounces/150 grams of baby broccoli
- 1 ounces/40 grams of raw Marcona almonds
- . three sprigs of fresh coriander
- 10 ½ ounces/300 grams of vegetable broth
- freshly ground black pepper
- sansho pepper
- lemongrass powder
- 3 ounces/75 grams of almond butter (see recipe)
- Salt
- extra virgin olive oil
- four radishes
- shichimi togarashi (optional)

STEPS

Clean the salmon loins and dry them well with absorbent paper, set aside. It will be cooked just before serving on a grill or in a non-stick pan, although those who prefer it can steam or bake it.

To prepare the cream, clean and chop the leek into not very thin slices and the smallest baby broccoli. This dish is a good option to take advantage of the broccoli stems that we saved from the chickpeas with the coconut milk recipe. Chop the fresh coriander leaves; you can also use the stems and vary the amount to taste; if you do not want its flavor to have much presence, you can reduce it.

Heat a large frying pan with a little extra virgin olive oil and add the leek, broccoli, raw almonds, chopped coriander, and season to taste. Saute over low heat for a few minutes until the vegetables begin to be tender. Then add the sansho pepper to the lemongrass powder, give it a couple of turns, add the broth and bring it to a boil. Cook for about five minutes.

Transfer the vegetables with the broth to the blender or Thermomix glass, add the almond butter and blend until you obtain a fine and homogeneous cream. Taste it in case it is necessary to rectify salt or spices.

Proceed to cook the fish, cook the salmon on the grill or in the pan, first on the skin side until crispy, then on the other side. Remember to add a little salt before cooking it.

Serve a base of almond cream and broccoli on the plates, place the salmon on top (if you want to preserve the crispy skin, it should be served upside down), a little radish sliced with the mandolin, and some baby broccoli tips. Add a little shichimi togarashi and a few extra virgin olive oil drops to the cream.

Salmon With Sesame And Orange, A Delicious And Easy Recipe For Air Fryer

Ingredients (4 people)

- four servings of fresh salmon
- 1 tsp of salt
- ½ tsp Japanese sansho pepper
- ½ tsp granulated garlic
- 2 tsp grated and dried orange peel
- 2-3 tsp raw white sesame
- 1 tsp toasted sesame oil
- 1 tablespoon of extra virgin olive oil.

STEPS

Clean and dry the salmon filets and season them with a little salt, the Japanese sansho pepper, and a pinch of granulated garlic. Then add the dried orange peel and add a little sesame oil.
Next, cover with the raw sesame seeds and press lightly so that they adhere. Finish with a little more toasted sesame oil and extra virgin olive oil.
Place the fish in a tray suitable for the air fryer and put it in the fryer, program 392°F/200° C and take about 8-10 minutes. Check the doneness in the first eight minutes, depending on your appliance and how you like the doneness of the salmon, extend the time or not.

Serve the salmon with sesame and orange on the plates accompanied by a little salad or the garnish you want, vegetables, rice, potatoes... To enhance its aroma and flavor, you can grate a little fresh orange peel and sprinkle a little shichimi togarashi.

Baked Sea Bass With Oyster Mushrooms And Pickled Lemon

Ingredients (4-6 people)

- one Corvina of 2 kg approx.
- two pickled lemons
- ½ head of garlic
- 18 ounces/500 grams of oyster mushrooms or gírgolas
- a few sprigs of fresh coriander
- 1 tsp of ground ñora
- ½ tsp ground white pepper
- 2 tablespoons of granulated almonds (optional)
- a pinch of salt
- 1 tbsp extra virgin olive oil.

STEPS

After descaling the Corvina, remove the head and spine of the Corvina and keep them to make broth; you can ask the fishmonger to do it, clean the fish to obtain the two whole loins. Turn on the oven to 392°F/200° C with heat up and down.
Drain the lemons from the government's liquid and cut them into quarters. Separate the garlic cloves and give them a blow to break; it is not necessary to remove the skin (in the shirt). Clean the mushrooms, and if they are very large, you can cut them roughly.
Arrange a bed of oyster mushrooms on the oven tray that you can cover with parchment paper, so it doesn't get so dirty. Place the sea bass filets on top and distribute the lemons, garlic, and fresh coriander sprigs.
Sprinkle the ground ñora, white pepper, and almonds, finally add salt to taste and a good

trickle of extra virgin olive oil. Put the tray in the oven and bake for about 18 minutes.
If you want the fish to brown a little more, raise the tray so that it is close to the grill and bake for four or five more minutes; the time may vary depending on the size of the Corvina pieces.
Serve the roasted Corvina portion with the mushrooms, the peeled garlic, and some fresh coriander leaves on the plates. You can add volume to the dish with a crispy leek nest.

Baked Sea Bass With Potatoes And Spring Garlic

Ingredients

- one wild sea bass of 1,800 kg
- 3-4 large new potatoes
- one bunch of tender garlic
- 8-10 large oyster mushrooms
- ½ glass of white wine (or a little more)
- 1 tbsp extra virgin olive oil
- a pinch of salt
- 1 tsp freshly ground pepper
- fresh curly parsley (optional)

STEPS

Peel the potatoes and cut them into slices to make them bakery-style, about half a centimeter thick. Peel the garlic cloves and leave them whole; chop a couple of them into small pieces to distribute them on the tray.
To speed up the cooking process of the potatoes, put them in a silicone case or a microwave-safe container and cook them in this small appliance for five minutes at maximum power. Another option is to fry the potatoes in plenty of olive oil without letting them brown.
Arrange the pre cooked potatoes on the oven tray to make a bed, cover them by distributing the oyster mushrooms and whole spring garlic and then place the sea bass that you will have previously cleaned (you can ask the fishmonger already clean) of scales and their interiors, without removing the head Season the sea bass to taste.
Add the white wine and a generous trickle of extra virgin olive oil, distribute the chopped spring garlic inside the sea bass and over the whole. Introduce the tray in the oven previously heated to 410°F/210° C with heat up and down and medium height. About 25 minutes of baking per kilo of fish are calculated, so we have approximately 40 minutes in this case.
In the last ten minutes, raise the tray a little so that it is closer to the grill and brown the skin of the sea bass; if necessary, remove the mushrooms because they will surely already be cooked.
To serve the baked sea bass, remove the skin and separate the head; the fish will easily release the central bone. Carefully and with the help of two fish serving spatulas, remove the filets and place them on the plate. Accompany with potatoes, mushrooms, and spring garlic. Garnish (optionally) with a few curly parsley leaves.

Mullets With Red Cabbage With Ginger And Sesame

Ingredients

- 4-8 red mullets (depending on size)
- ½ medium red cabbage
- three garlic cloves
- one piece of ginger root (about the size of a walnut)
- 2 cup /260ml mushroom broth (you can use vegetable broth)
- ½ tsp ground cumin
- black pepper
- black sesame seeds
- extra virgin olive oil
- Sesame oil
- Salt.

STEPS

Cut the red cabbage into julienne strips, pour a good splash of olive oil into a large frying pan, add the seasoned cabbage to taste; fry for a few minutes, and add the minced garlic cloves and the peeled. Grated ginger, let it Brown, stirring occasionally, and pour in the mushroom broth, cumin, and freshly ground black pepper. Bring to a boil and cook over medium or high heat, depending on how tender you want the red cabbage.

Remove the loins from the red mullet, salt them to taste, and grill them in a frying pan with a little oil, first on the skin side, then turn them over. Meanwhile, in another ungreased pan, toast the sesame seeds.

Mix two tablespoons of extra virgin olive oil and one tablespoon of sesame oil and transfer to the plating.

Serve the red cabbage with ginger in the center of the plate, place the red mullet with the black sesame on it, finally water the whole with a teaspoon of olive oil and sesame.

Salad Of Verdinas, Prawns, And Spinach

Ingredients

- 18 ounces/500 grams of cooked green beans
- 14 ounces/400 grams of cherry tomatoes
- one clove garlic
- 24 prawns
- one head of lettuce
- 7 ounces/200 grams spinach sprouts
- one avocado
- ½ red onion
- a handful of black olives
- one tablespoon of sweet corn
- a pinch of salt
- 1 tbsp candied tomato oil

STEPS

Drain the verdins from their cooking water; if you buy them already cooked, rinse them by putting them in a strainer and under running water from the tap. Booking.

Wash and dry the cherry tomatoes, peel the garlic clove and cut it half. Heat a grill with a little extra virgin olive oil and sauté the tomatoes with the garlic for a couple of minutes, and that's it.

Peel the prawns or prawns, reserve the heads and carcasses to make a broth or sauce and on the same grill, cook the bodies with a little extra virgin olive oil and salt to taste. Make them very little so that they are juicy.

Strip the bud and wash the leaves, drain them well and chop them. Wash (if necessary) the spinach sprouts and drain well. Cut, pit, and peel the avocado and cut it into slices. Peel the red onion and finely chop it.

Serve the legume and prawn salad in small bowls or deep plates; first place the lettuce and spinach and then harmoniously arrange the green vegetables, sautéed tomatoes, prawns, avocado, and red onion. Also, accompany the black olives and sweet corn, and to finish, season with the candied tomato oil and a few flakes of salt.

Mediterranean Boneless

Ingredients
- one boneless chicken thigh
- one chicken breast
- eight pineapple slices
- one large bag of mixed salad or mesclun
- four radishes
- ½ Granny Smith apple
- four hanging tomatoes
- ½ purple onion
- one large avocado
- a handful of dried fruit
- 1 tbsp extra virgin olive oil
- 1 pinch of salt.

For the dressing
- 2 tbsp of raw honey
- 2 tbsp of lime juice
- 2 tbsp of soy sauce
- 1-2 tsp sriracha sauce
- three tbsp of extra virgin olive oil
- a pinch of salt

STEPS

In the ingredients, there is a high and a chicken breast, but it can also be made with just the thighs or just with the breasts of this bird. To begin with, you have to cut the meat into cubes less than bite-size to combine it with other elements of the salad.

Put a drizzle of extra virgin olive oil in a pan and sauté the chicken until golden brown, then remove and set aside. In the same pan, grill the pineapple slices; if you don't have natural pineapple, you can use the preserve, but not in syrup, pineapple in its juice (no added sugar). When the pineapple has browned on both sides, remove it and reserve.

Wash and drain the lettuce or mesclun leaves, wash the radishes, cut the two ends, and then cut them into very thin slices. Wash the apple and without peeling it, cut it into thin sticks. Wash the tomatoes and cut them in half or quarters; if you don't have hanging tomatoes, you can put two cherry tomatoes per plate. Peel the red onion and cut it into julienne strips.

The last ingredient to prepare is the avocado to prevent it from turning black. Cut it in half, and then in quarters, remove the bone and skin, and cut slices or cubes, as you like. Prepare the dressing by mixing the honey, lime juice, soy sauce, sriracha sauce, extra virgin olive oil, and salt; you can do it in a bowl or a jar with a lid, shaking it like a cocktail shaker, until it emulsifies the sauce. Serve a base of assorted lettuce on each plate, arrange a row of sautéed chicken in the center, place the grilled pineapple slices on one side, and distribute the avocado and tomato on one side or both sides of the chicken. On the meat, alternately place the radishes and the green apple, and to finish, distribute the chopped nuts. Dress the salad with the special sauce of sriracha, soy, and honey at the table.

Lentil, Smoked Salmon And Avocado Salad

Ingredients

- 18 ounces/500 grams of cooked lentils
- one bag of arugula
- four radishes
- 8 ounces/225 grams of smoked salmon
- one avocado
- 1 tsp black or white sesame seeds
- a pinch of salt
- 1 tbsp of extra virgin olive oil
- 1 tbsp of apple cider vinegar (optional).

STEPS

If you have to cook the lentils and need a recipe to follow step by step, you can go to the recipe for lentils with asparagus and strawberries indicated at the beginning of this post; you can also see this recipe for lentils for Thermomix. In any case, prepare them in time to cool down. If you use canned lentils, transfer them to a strainer and rinse them under running water.

Prepare the arugula leaves and the radishes, cut them into thin slices, and then into sticks. Cut the salmon into not very thin strips or small cubes; think about how you will enjoy the salad more if you find a piece of this oily fish in each bite or just from time to time. Cut the avocado into quarters, remove the stone and skin, and cut it into small cubes. In the meantime, you can toast the sesame seeds in an ungreased pan to enhance their flavor.

To dress this legume salad with avocado and salmon, you can make a vinaigrette with extra virgin olive oil, a little apple cider vinegar, and salt, but it also goes very well with just a good EVOO and a little salt. And if you have fresh chopped chives, it works great.

Serve the salad, the arugula, the lentils, the radishes, the smoked salmon, and the sesame seeds on the plates; you can do it harmoniously or simply by mixing it in a bowl beforehand. Season to taste with a little salt and a good extra virgin olive oil to finish.

Bean Salad With Avocado, Tomato And Sweet And Sour Radishes

Ingredients

- 14 ounces/300-400 grams of cooked white beans
- 5 ounces/150 grams of red onion
- 5 ounces /150 grams of zucchini
- 15-20 cherry tomatoes
- 2 avocados
- 7 ounces /200 grams of sweet and sour radishes
- a few cubes of Iberian ham (omit in vegetarian diets)
- a few stalks of chives
- freshly ground black pepper
- Salt
- extra virgin olive oil.

STEPS

Cook white beans ahead of time to cool them down or choose quality canned (or bulk) cooked beans. If they are a preserve, wash them well to remove the government liquid. Reserve the beans and prepare the rest of the ingredients.

Peel the onion and finely chop it. Wash the zucchini well and cut it into small cubes; they will add a crunchy and fresh texture to the salad and a mild flavor. Wash the cherry or cocktail tomatoes and cut them in half.

The avocados should be prepared when all the mise en place is ready to be placed on the plate immediately after pearling and cut and prevent them from oxidizing. And the pickled radishes must be made at least the day before

To make the avocado rose for this salad, you can follow the instructions in the video in this post. However, if you don't want to be entertained, you can cut the avocado into small cubes and spread it over the salad with the rest of the ingredients.

Put the white beans in a bowl and add the spring onion, courgette, and cherry tomatoes; add a few Iberian ham cubes. Season with freshly ground black pepper, salt, and extra virgin olive oil. Mix well. Arrange the avocado rose in the center of the plate, serve the bean salad around it and surround it with the sweet and sour radish slices. Chop the chives and spread them over the plate, and to finish, pour a trickle of extra virgin olive oil.

Tasty Beef and Broccoli

Ingredients
- 1 ½ pounds flanks steak, cut into thin strips
- 1 tablespoon olive oil
- 1 tablespoon tamari sauce
- 1 cup beef stock
- 450 g /1 pound broccoli, florets separated

STEPS

In a bowl, mix steak strips with oil and tamari, toss and leave aside for 10 minutes. Set your instant pot on sauté mode, add beef strips and brown them for 4 minutes on each side.

Add stock, stir, cover pot again and cook on high for 8 minutes.
Add broccoli, stir, cover pot again and cook on high for 4 minutes more.
Divide everything between plates and serve.

Beef Corn Chili

Ingredients
- 2 small onions, chopped (finely)
- ¼ cup canned corn
- 1 tablespoon oil
- 10 ounces/ 300g lean ground beef
- 2 small chili peppers, diced

STEPS

Take your instant pot and place over dry kitchen surface; open its top lid and switch it on.
Press. "SAUTE".
In its Cooking pot, add and heat the oil.
Add the onions, chili pepper, and beef; cook for 2-3 minutes until turn translucent and softened.
Add the 3 cups water in the Cooking pot; combine to mix well.
Close its top lid and make sure that its valve it closed to avoid spilling.
Press "MEAT/STEW". Adjust the timer to 20 minutes.
Press will slowly build up; let the added ingredients to cook until the timer indicates zero.
Press "CANCEL". Now press "NPR" for natural release pressure. Instant pot will gradually release pressure for about 8-10 minutes.
Open the top lid; transfer the cooked recipe in serving plates.
Serve the recipe warm.

Balsamic Beef Dish

Ingredients

- 3 pounds chuck roast
- 3 cloves garlic, thinly sliced
- 1 tablespoon oil
- 1 teaspoon flavored vinegar
- ½ teaspoon pepper
- ½ teaspoon rosemary
- 1 tablespoon butter
- ½ teaspoon thyme
- ¼ cup balsamic vinegar
- 1 cup beef broth

STEPS

Cut slits in the roast and stuff garlic slices all over.
Take a bowl and add flavored vinegar, rosemary, pepper, thyme and rub the mixture over the roast.
Set your pot to sauté mode and add oil, allow the oil to heat up.
Add roast and brown both sides (5 minutes each side).
Take the roast out and keep it on the side.
Add butter, broth, balsamic vinegar and deglaze the pot.
Transfer the roast back and lock up the lid, cook on HIGH pressure for 40 minutes.
Perform a quick release.
Remove the lid and serve!

Soy Sauce Beef Roast

Ingredients

- ½ teaspoon beef bouillon
- 1 ½ teaspoon rosemary
- ½ teaspoon minced garlic
- 900 g /2 pounds roast beef
- 1/3 cup soy sauce

STEPS

Mix the soy sauce, bouillon, rosemary, and garlic together in a mixing bowl.
Place your instant pot over as dry kitchen platform. Open the top lid and plug it on.
Add the roast, bowl mix and enough water to cover the roast; gently stir to mix well.
Properly close the top lid; make sure that the safety valve is properly locked.
Press "MEAT/STEW" Cooking function; set pressure level to "HIGH" and set the Cooking time to 35 minutes.
Allow the pressure to build to cook the ingredients.
After Cooking time is over press "CANCEL" setting. Find and press "NPR" Cooking function. This setting is for the natural release of inside pressure, and it takes around 10 minutes to slowly release pressure.
Slowly open the lid, take out the cooked meat and shred it.
Add the shredded meat back in the potting mix and stir to mix well.
Take out the cooked recipe in serving containers. Serve warm.

Rosemary Beef Chuck Roast

Ingredients

- 3 pounds / 1,300 kg chuck beef roast
- 3 garlic cloves
- ¼ cup balsamic vinegar
- 1 sprig fresh rosemary
- 1 sprig fresh thyme
- 1 cup of water
- 1 tablespoon vegetable oil
- Salt and pepper to taste

STEPS

Cut slices in the beef roast and place the garlic cloves in them.
Coat the roast with the herbs, black pepper, and salt.
Preheat your instant pot using the sauté setting and add the oil.
When warmed, add the beef roast and stir-cook until browned on all sides.
Add the remaining ingredients; stir gently.
Seal the lid and cook on high pressure for 40 minutes using the manual setting.
Let the pressure release naturally, about 10 minutes.
Uncover the instant pot; transfer the beef roast the serving plates, slice and serve.

Pork Chops and Tomato Sauce

Ingredients

- 4 pork chops, boneless
- 1 tablespoon soy sauce
- ¼ teaspoon sesame oil
- 1 ½ cups tomato paste
- 1 yellow onion
- 8 mushrooms, sliced

STEPS

In a bowl, mix pork chops with soy sauce and sesame oil, toss and leave aside for 10 minutes.
Set your instant pot on sauté mode, add pork chops and brown them for 5 minutes on each side.
Add onion, stir and cook for 1-2 minutes more.
Add tomato paste and mushrooms, toss, cover and cook on high for 8-9 minutes.
Divide everything between plates and serve.

Pork Potato

Ingredients

- 10 ounces / 300g pork neck, fat remove and make small pieces
- 1 medium sweet potato, chopped
- 1 tablespoon oil
- 3 cups beef stock, Low – sodium
- 1 onion, chopped (finely)

STEPS

Take your pot and place over dry kitchen surface; open its top lid and switch it on. Press "sauté". Grease the pot with some Cooking oil.
Add the onions; cook for 2 minutes until turn translucent and softened.
Add the meat; stir-cook for 4-5 minutes to evenly brown.
Mix in the stock and potatoes.
Close its top lid and make sure that its valve it closed to avoid spillage.

Press "Manual". Adjust the timer to 20 minutes.
Pressure will slowly build up; let the added ingredients to cook until the timer indicates zero.
Press "CANCEL". Now press "NPR" for natural release pressure. Instant pot will gradually release pressure for about 8-10 minutes.

Pasta Carbonara

Ingredients

- 1 packet spaghetti
- 3 ½ ounces/100 g bacon (cut in strips)
- 3 Eggs
- 1 Egg yolk
- 3 ½ ounces/100 gpecorino romano or parmesan, grated
- 1 tbsp olive oil
- Black pepper (coarsely crushed)
- Salt to taste

STEPS

In a large pan or a saucepan, heat the olive oil and fry the bacon till crisp. Set aside.
In a mixing bowl, beat the whole eggs and the yollk well. Stir in the grated cheese and set aside.
Boil the spaghetti in abundant salty water. Drain the pasta, reserving some of the cooking water.
In another saucepan, toss the pasta with the egg mixture, bacon and any fat rendered from cooking the bacon, over very low heat. Make sure that the individual strands of pasta are all coated properly with the mixture. Season with salt, add the pasta water, give it a quick toss, and remove right away from the heat.
The sauce should have a creamy texture, which will be lost if the pasta remains on the fire for too long.
The idea is to cook the egg with the heat of the pasta, and not with the heat of the fire.
Serve right away with lots of pepper, freshly crushed in a pepper mill, and more Parmesan if desired.

Margherita Pizza

Ingredients

For Pizza dough:
- 18 ounces /500 g flour
- Salt
- 10 ounces /300 ml tepid Water
- ½ tbsp /7 g dried yeast
- ½ tsp sugar
- 2 tbsp/30 ml olive oil
- Extra virgin olive oil

For the topping:
- Passata sauce
- 1 cup Mozzarella cheese, grated
- Handful of basil leaves
- Pepper
- Extra virgin olive oil

STEPS

Sieve flour with salt and add yeast to tepid water and stir in sugar. Leave aside for 6 to 8 minutes.
In a mixing bowl, create a well in the middle of the flour mixture and add 3 ounces /100 ml of yeast mixture and 0,5 ounce /15 ml olive oil.

Add in the rest of yeast mixture and remaining olive oil.
Flour the kneading surface so that the dough does not stick.
Mix together with your fingers till you have a dough. Knead for 10 minutes till you have an elastic, even product.

Proving the Dough

Place the dough in a bowl and drizzle generously with extra virgin olive oil.
Cover bowl with cling film and place in a warm area to prove for 50 minutes.
After the dough is proved, bash the air out and cut into small pieces for individual pizzas.
Dust the work surface and rolling pin with some flour before rolling out the dough.

Preparing the Topping

Pre-heat oven at its highest mark and flour your baking tray.
Now, using a rolling pin, roll out the freshly made pizza dough and place on the tray.
Spread a thin layer of passata sauce and cover with mozarella cheese and sprinkle basil leaves.
Put the tray into the oven for 10 to 12 minutes
After the pizza is baked remove from the oven and drizzle extra virgin olive oil and some pepper.
Garnish with fresh basil and cut into slices.

Mushroom Risotto

Ingredients

- 1 Tbsp Olive oil
- 2 tbsp / 25 g Butter
- 1 Onion, chopped
- 7 ounces /200 g Mushrooms, sliced
- ½ cup Arborio rice
- ¼ cup White wine (optional)
- 4 cups Hot chicken stock/veg stock
- 1/3 cup Parmesan cheese, grated
- 1 tbsp Parsley
- 2 tbsp/25 g Extra butter just before serving
- Salt
- Pepper

STEPS

Saute onion and mushrooms in oil and butter until soft.
Stir in rice and cook till transparent, add wine if it gets dry.
Stir in 1 ladle of stock. Stir well, cover and simmer gently for several minutes or till rice looks dry.
Add more stock, stir, cover and keep repeating this process till rice is just cooked (about 25 minutes).
Taste and add a little salt.
Now remove from heat and stir in parmesan, parsley, extra butter if using and pepper to taste.

Pasta Con Pomodoro E Basilico

Ingredients

- 35 ounces /1 Kg red ripe tomatoes, large
- 3 tbsp/40 ml extra virgin olive oil
- 3 garlic cloves (minced), peeled
- Handful fresh basil
- A pinch of red chilly flakes
- 1 packet penne (though you could use any pasta here, long, thin, short or tube, as this is a sauce which works well with all the pastas
- parmesan cheeseto taste
- Salt

STEPS

Cut the tomatoes in half crosswise and remove most of the seeds, using your fingers. Then quarter the tomatoes.
Heat the oil in a large skillet, and add garlic and chilly flakes.
As soon as the garlic gives off its aroma and becomes opaque, add the tomatoes. Cook over high heat until the tomato begins to thicken. Use a wooden spoon to stir and help break the tomato pulp.
Add the basil, either whole or roughly chopped, and salt. When the sauce is cooked, remove it from the heat and run it through a food processor for a minute.
Cook the pasta in abundant boiling water, till al dente, and drain.
Place in a serving bowl with the sauce.
Drizzle a little olive oil over the pasta and mix well with the sauce.
Serve with grated Parmesan cheese.

Fettuccine Pomodoro

Ingredients

- 14 ounces /400 g Fettucine pasta, blanched
- 10 tbsp/150 Ml Olive oil
- 1 tbsp/18 gOnion, chopped
- 1 tbsp/ 15gGarlic, chopped
- 24 ounces /700g Roma tomato (diced)
- ¼ tbsp /5 g Red pepper flakes
- 1 ¼ tbsp/20 gFresh basil
- 4 tbsp /60g Butter, unsalted
- ½ tbsp/8 gDried olive powder

STEPS

Heat oil in a large skillet over medium-low flame.
Cook onion, stirring occasionally, until soft, 10–12 minutes.
Add garlic and cook, stirring, about 3 minutes.
Add red pepper flakes and cook, stirring for a minute.
Increase heat to medium, add puréed tomatoes, and season lightly with salt.
Cook, stirring occasionally, until sauce thickens slightly and flavors have come together, 20–25 minutes. Remove from heat and stir in basil.
Set skillet over high heat and stir in reserved pasta cooking liquid to loosen sauce; bring to a boil.
Add pasta and cook, stirring, until sauce coats pasta and pasta is al dente.
Serve garnished with fresh basil sprig and olive powder.

Classic Pasta Amatriciana

Ingredients

- 2 Tbsp extra virgin olive oil
- 2 tbsp /30g butter, unsalted
- ½ cup /150g pancetta or bacon (diced)
- 1 Onion (diced)
- 6-8 Garlic cloves (minced)
- 2 tbsp tomato paste
- 8-10 Tomatoes (riped), chopped

For garnishing:
- Cherry tomatoes
- Olives
- Ham (optional)
- 3 tbsp /50g parmigiano-reggiano cheese (plus more for serving), grated
- Salt
- 2 tbsp parsley
- 12 ounces /350g dried Fusili pasta or any type available
- 1 tbsp dried herbs (thyme , rosemary, oregano)

STEPS

Heat the olive oil in a large skillet over medium heat. Add the diced bacon and cook, stirring frequently, until most of the fat has rendered into the pan and the bacon is crispy and caramelized slightly.
Add the diced onion and saute in the rendered fat for 3 to 5 minutes, stirring frequently, until the onions are soft and lightly caramelized.
Add the garlic and continue to saute for an addition 2 to 3 minutes, being careful to avoid burning the garlic or onion. Deglaze the pan with a tablespoon of water or red wine (optional), to remove any bits of crispy pancetta or bits from the bottom of the pan.
Add the tomato paste and the dried herbs and continue to cook, stirring frequently, over medium heat for an addition 1 to 2 minutes, or until the paste has thickened slightly.
Add the tomatoes,bring the sauce to a low simmer, and cook, stirring every few minutes, for 15 to 20 minutes. The sauce should be relatively thick and season to taste with salt. Place over low heat while you cook the pasta.

Meanwhile, bring a large pot of salted water to boil.
Add the pasta and cook until al-dente.
Reserve 1/2 to 3/4 cup of the pasta cooking water in a measuring cup,
and then drain the pasta.
Return the drained pasta back into the pot, add the sauce, thinning with past cooking water as necessary until the pasta is evenly coated.
Serve pasta with a topping of cherry tomatoes,
olives ,extra virgin olive oil
and some grated Parmigiano-Reggiano cheese .

CHAPTER 8

Snacks And Sides

Recipes

Tomato, Avocado, Egg And Sweet And Sour Cucumber Sandwich

Ingredients

- one bagel of seeds and cereals
- 1 tbsp of fresh cheese to spread
- two thin slices of tomato
- ½ avocado
- 1 hard-boiled egg
- ½ cucumber, sweet and sour onion
- a pinch of salt.

STEPS

The hard-boiled egg can be ready in ten minutes; you know that its cooking should not exceed 8 minutes so that the yolk does not remain green and very dry; once the egg is cooked, it can be cooled with water before peeling it.

The sweet and sour cucumber will have to be prepared in advance; here is the recipe for sweet and sour cucumber. Prepared with these ingredients, we go with the simple elaboration of the sandwich.

Wash the tomato that you are going to use well; in this case, it is a salad tomato, and for the size of the roll, two thin slices are enough (they overlap slightly). Peel the avocado and cut it into slices.
Open the bread in half, spread the two halves with the fresh cheese, place the tomato on the base of the sandwich with cheese, and then place the avocado covering it completely. Then place four thin slices of hard-boiled egg and add a pinch of salt. Cover the egg with cucumber and sweet and sour onion, and cover again with a hard-boiled egg. Cover the sandwich with the top of the bread, and that's it.

White Bean And Bacon Dip

Ingredients
- 12 ounces /350 gof cooked white beans
- 3 ½ ounces /100 g of meat broth
- one clove garlic
- 1 tsp grated lemon peel
- 1 tsp harissa sauce
- 2 tbsp/30 g of Parmesan
- black pepper

- Salt
- 8 slices of bacon
- chive
- extra virgin olive oil

STEPS

Once you have the cooked beans, put them in the blender jar well-drained. Add the broth, the previously peeled clove of garlic, and remove the germ from inside.

Grate the skin of the lemon and incorporate it, also add the harissa sauce (if not, you can add another spicy chili sauce), the parmesan cut into pieces (chopping or crushing it will leave small lumps that are very pleasant to taste), a pinch of salt and black pepper. Blend until creamy and taste to rectify salt, pepper, or hot sauce.

Heat a frying pan without adding any oil, and cook the bacon slices until crispy. You may be interested in remembering how to make crispy bacon with less fat. When it's done, cut it with scissors.

Reserve a couple of tablespoons of bacon and add the rest to the cream of beans, mix well and pour it into a bowl that is comfortable to eat.

Top the dip with the reserved bacon, add the chopped chives, and finish with a good trickle of extra virgin olive oil. Accompany the white bean dip with pita bread, naan bread, tortillas, toast, breadsticks, crudités…

Avocado, Mozzarella, And Roasted Pepper
Pate Sandwich

Ingredients

- 8 slices of sliced bread (or whatever you prefer)
- 8 tablespoons roasted pepper pâté (see recipe)
- 2 balls of fresh mozzarella
- 2 large avocados
- a pinch of freshly ground black pepper
- 1 tsp extra virgin olive oil.

STEPS

Start by lightly toasting the bread on a grill lightly greased with extra virgin olive oil, but toast them only on one side, the one that will be on the outside, so that the bread's tender interior will absorb the pate of peppers very well.

Drain the fresh mozzarella balls from the government liquid and cut them into slices; if they are small pieces, you may need some more.

Cut the avocados to remove the stone and peel them, then cut them into not very thin slices so that it is in balance with the cheese and the rest of the ingredients.

Spread the slices of bread with a plate of roasted peppers, putting a little more on the slice that will be the base than on the one that will be the top of the sandwich.

Place the bread base with vegetable pate on the plate, then arrange the slices of fresh mozzarella and then the avocado with a little freshly ground black pepper. Serve right away.

Ham And Brie Cheese Piadina

Ingredients

- 4 piadinas
- 8 slices of serrano ham
- some lettuce leaves
- 2 large red tomatoes
- one portion of brie cheese

- extra virgin olive oil
- chive
- freshly ground black pepper
- salt.

STEPS

Start by preparing the dressing, put the extra virgin olive oil you need to dress the vegetables in the blender glass, add chopped fresh chives, black pepper, and salt, grind lightly, leaving some stems of whole chives. Booking.

Wash the lettuce leaves and drain or dry them well. Wash the tomatoes and cut them into thin slices. Cut the brie cheese into strips lengthwise and then two or three pieces. Start assembling the piadina.

Place two rolled slices of ham in the middle of the bread, place a little lettuce and tomato on top of the ham, dress with the chive oil, place the cheese, and if you wish, slightly heat the Piadina with ham and brie cheese, carefully that it does not affect the lettuce, one option is to bring the kitchen torch to low power. Finish with one more string of chive dressing and serve right away.

Crispy And Spicy Chickpeas

Ingredients

- 14 ounces /400 g of cooked chickpeas
- 1 tsp salt
- 2 tsp paprika from La Vera
- 1 tsp cumin powder
- 1 tsp onion powder
- 1 tsp grated garlic powder
- 1 tsp black pepper
- 1 tsp turmeric rasa
- 1-2 tsp dried coriander leaves
- 1 tablespoon of extra virgin olive oil.

STEPS

You can use canned chickpeas to make this recipe, pour them into a large colander and rinse them under running tap water until they stop foaming. Drain them well and transfer them to a container covered with kitchen paper or a cloth to dry them.

Next, transfer the chickpeas to a bowl, add the salt, spices, and extra virgin olive oil, mix well, and put them in the air fryer basket; you can cover it with parchment paper to make it less dirty.

Program 200° C for about nine minutes; this is the time we put with the chubby chickpeas; smaller varieties can reduce the time. Our air fryer is around 2,000 watts of power; the time may vary for other fryers with less power.

When the chickpeas are crispy and toasted, transfer them to a tray to cool. It is possible that some of them have burst, but they can be eaten anyway. You can keep this snack in a closed jar to have it on hand whenever you feel like it.

Carrot Chips

Ingredients

- 5 large carrots (if possible organic)
- a pinch of salt
- a pinch of freshly ground black pepper.

STEPS

Wash the carrots, peel them with a vegetable peeler, and cut them very thin with the mandolin. You can make the cuts as you like, round or elongated, although it is better if they are a little long as their size is reduced.

Regarding the number of carrots that should be made per person, since it depends on how much you want to eat, think that the carrot is mostly water, so when you extract it, turn it into a crunchy snack, practically all the volume is lost. If you eat only one carrot raw, dehydrated, you could eat three or more.

Cover a microwave-safe plate with parchment paper and place the thin slices of carrot, season with salt and pepper, put it in the microwave, and program for about five or six minutes at 800 watts, checking from time to time if they change color. When they start to brown, remove the carrot from the microwave and transfer the chips, which won't be quite crisp, to a wire rack. When they cool, they will be crispy.

Cherry-Peach Compote with Greek Yogurt

Ingredients

- 4 peaches, halved, pitted, and thinly sliced
- 450 g/1 lb. cherries, pitted and halved
- 2 cups red wine
- ¾ cup coconut sugar
- 1 ½ cups Greek yogurt

What you'll need from the store cupboard:
- 1 tsp cinnamon powder
- 1 tsp vanilla extract
- 1 tbsp date syrup

STEPS

In a medium bowl, combine peaches, cherries, and cinnamon. Toss and set aside. In a medium saucepan, mix the red wine with coconut sugar, and heat over medium heat until the sugar dissolves and mixture syrupy, 5 minutes. Stir frequently.
Pour the hot syrup over the fruits and set aside to cool for 1 hour.
In another medium bowl, combine the Greek yogurt, vanilla, and date syrup. Plate the fruits and top with generous dollops of the yogurt mixture.
Serve.

Roasted Peach and Orange Crostini

Ingredients

- 1/3 cup Greek yogurt
- 230g /8 oz cream cheese, room temperature
- 3 peaches, pitted and thinly sliced
- 1 orange, 3 tbsp of juice
- 8 slices whole-grain baguette, toasted

What you'll need from the store cupboard:
- 1/3 cup coconut sugar
- a pinch cinnamon powder
- a pinch nutmeg powder
- 1 tbsp date syrup for drizzling

STEPS

In a food processor, add the yogurt, cream cheese, coconut sugar, cinnamon, and nutmeg. Process until well blended. Transfer mixture to a bowl, cover with a plastic wrap and refrigerate for 1 hour.
Preheat the oven to 425 F and line a baking sheet with parchment paper. Set aside.
In a bowl, add the peaches and drizzle with the orange juice. Toss and transfer the peaches to the baking sheet. Roast in the oven until the peaches are tender, 20 to 25 minutes.

After, arrange the toasted bread (crostini) on a clean flat surface, spread with the Greek yogurt, and share the peaches on top. Drizzle with the date syrup.
Plate and serve.

Pumpkin Yogurt Parfait

Ingredients

- 1 (15 oz) can pumpkin puree
- 1 ¼ cup Greek yogurt
- A handful of walnuts for garnishing

What you'll need from the store cupboard:
- 1 tsp vanilla extract
- 2 tbsp date syrup
- 2 ½ tbsp coconut sugar
- a pinch nutmeg powder
- 2 tsp cinnamon powder

STEPS

In a medium bowl, combine the pumpkin puree, yogurt, vanilla, date syrup, coconut sugar, nutmeg, and cinnamon. Puree using an immersion blender until smooth. Adjust the taste with more coconut sugar as desired. Divide the mixture into serving glasses and refrigerate for 20 to 30 minutes.
Remove from the fridge, top with the walnuts, and drizzle with more date syrup as desired.
Serve immediately.

Chocolate-Coated Dates

Ingredients

- 16 dates
- 16 pecans, toasted
- 1 ½ cups unsweetened chocolate chips
- 1 tbsp shelled pistachios, crushed
- 1 tbsp desiccated coconut

What you'll need from the store cupboard:
- 2 tsp date syrup
  1 tsp extra virgin olive oil
- 1 tsp cinnamon powder

STEPS

Line a baking sheet with parchment paper and set aside.
Cut a slit in the dates, remove the pits, and replace with a pecan each. Close up the dates and set aside.
In a medium safe microwave bowl, add the chocolate, date syrup, olive oil, and cinnamon. Microwave for 1 minute while stirring at every 10-second interval until the chocolate melts completely.
Remove the bowl and coat each date in the chocolate mixture.
Arrange the dates on the baking tray and sprinkle with the pistachios and coconut.
Freeze for 1 hour, remove and leave at room temperature for 10 minutes.
Serve and enjoy!

Cashew and Peanut Rice Pudding

Ingredients

- 2 cups 2 % skimmed milk
- 1 cup heavy cream
- 1 cup brown rice, rinsed
- 1/3 cup organic evaporated milk
- 1/2 cup toasted cashews and walnuts, crushed

What you'll need from the store cupboard:
- 2 tsp vanilla extract
- 2 tsp cinnamon powder
- 3 tbsp granulated sugar
- 2 tbsp grass-fed butter, room temperature
- Date syrup for topping

STEPS

In a large pot, combine the skimmed milk, heavy cream, vanilla, and cinnamon. Heat over medium temperature and just when about boiling, remove from the fire and set aside to cool completely.
Stir in the rice, sugar, and 1 cup of water. Bring to a boil over medium heat and then simmer for 30 to 40 minutes while stirring regularly.
Add more water as the liquid on the rice dries out with frequent stirring until the rice is moist and fully cooked, 10 to 15 minutes. Turn off the heat and stir in the butter and evaporated milk until well combined.
Dish the pudding into serving bowls, top with some date syrup, the cashews, and peanuts.
Serve immediately or chilled.

Apple Crisp

Ingredients

- 1/4 Cup Brown Sugar
- 1 Cup Rolled Oats
- 1 Tablespoon Maple Syrup
- 2 Teaspoons Cinnamon
- 5 Apples, Cut into Chunks

STEPS

Place all your ingredients into your instant pot, and then pour in a half a cup of water. Add in a pinch of salt.
Mix well, and then seal your instant pot. Cook on high pressure for eight minutes, and then allow for a natural pressure release. Allow it to sit for five minutes so the sauce has time to thicken before serving warm or room temperature.

White Bean Dip

Ingredients

- 850 g/30 Ounces Cannellini Beans, Rinsed & Drained
- 2 Cloves Garlic
- 1/4 Cup Olive Oil
- 1/4 Cup Vegetable Stock
- 1 Teaspoon Italian Seasoning

STEPS

Start by adding your vegetable stock and beans into your instant pot, and then press the chili function.
When the time is up, allow for a natural pressure release.

Transfer this into the blender, and then add in your remaining ingredients.
Blend until smooth, and serve with bread or crackers.

Grilled Flatbread with Burrata Cheese

Ingredients

- 18 oz/ 500 g cherry tomatoes
- olive oil
- kosher salt
- freshly ground pepper
- 4 skewers used for grilling
- Flatbread
- 450 g/1 lb fresh pizza dough
- flour for dusting
- ¾ cup olive oil
- 220 g /8 oz burrata cheese, drained in a colander
- 220 g /8 oz parmesan cheese, grated
- 2 tbsp fresh basil, chopped

STEPS

Divide the tomatoes evenly and pierce them with the skewers. Pour a small amount of olive oil over each skewer, sprinkle with salt and pepper.
Turn grill on. Over low heat, lay tomato Skewers in the center of the grill. Grill for 5-10 minutes rotating ½ way through.
While tomatoes are on the grill prepare flatbread dough. Start by cutting the pound of dough in 4 equal parts. Using flour, roll each portion of dough into ¼ inch thickness. Using a pastry brush, coat one side of the dough with a generous amount of olive oil. Take tomatoes off grill and place dough oil side down on grill. Carefully coat the other side of dough with oil. When large bubbles start forming on top side of dough, flip dough using a metal spatula. After flipping dough, sprinkle parmesan cheese evenly over all four flatbreads. Carefully take burrata cheese out of the colander, and pull small pieces off, placing them evenly over the four grilled flatbreads. Cover the grill lid for a few mins to let the cheese melt a little.
Take flatbread off the grill and sprinkle with basil. Serve with tomato skewers.

Fruicuterie Board

Ingredients

- 4 ounces/ 110 g blue cheese, such as Danish Blue
- 4 ounces/ 110 g aged goat cheese, such as Cypress Grove Midnight Moon
- 4 ounces / 110g Brie, such as President Brie
- 4 ounces/110 g soft triple crème cheese, such as Fromagerie Germain
- 4 ounces / 110 g Cotswold cheese
- 3 kiwis, peeled and thickly sliced
- 3 golden kiwis, peeled and thickly sliced
- 2 mangoes, peeled and diced
- 4 small bunches of grapes
- 4 handfuls of cherries
- 8 figs, quartered
- 2 peaches, thickly sliced
- 2 white peaches, thickly sliced
- 3 apricots, thickly sliced
- 3 plums, thickly sliced
- 1 cup cubed watermelon
- 1 cup cubed cantaloupe
- 1 cup halved strawberries
- 1 cup blackberries
- 1 cup raspberries
- 1 cup golden raspberries

STEPS

Place the cheeses on a large platter and let them sit at room temperature for 20 to 30 minutes until softened. Arrange the fruit in clusters around the cheese.

Baked Beet Chips

Ingredients

- 6-8 medium to large beets
- Olive oil
- 1 tablespoon flaked sea salt
- 1 tablespoon dried chives

STEPS

Trim the beets of greens and the roots. Scrub the beets well under cold water, but leave the skins on. Use a mandoline to slice the beets 1/16" thin. If you don't have a mandoline, use a very sharp knife to thinly slice the beets.

Preheat the oven to 400° F. Drizzle a very scant amount of olive oil to a baking sheet pan, then rub the oil over the pan with your hands or a paper towel. You want this to be a very scant layer, just enough so the beets don't stick, but not enough so they cook in the oil or they will steam instead of bake and come out limp instead of crisp. Layer the sliced beets onto the pan being careful not to overlap. You will need more than one sheet pan, and/or reuse the pans in batches of baking.

Bake the chips on the bottom rack of the oven for 10-15 minutes, depending on how thin the beets are cut and how large they are. While the beets are baking, pour the salt into a small bowl and crush the dried chives into the salt. You could do this step ahead of time as the longer the herbs are in the salt, the more flavorful the salt becomes.

Remove the rack from the oven and sprinkle with the chive salt. Allow the beets to cool on the pan, they'll crisp as they cool. Once cool, transfer to a cooling rack to continue to dry and crisp. Repeat with the remaining slices of beets.

Smoked Salmon and Avocado Summer Rolls

Ingredients
- 12 round rice paper wrappers
- 6 smoked salmon slices
- 1 avocado, thinly sliced
- 2-3 cups raw sprouts or cooked vermicelli
- 1 english cucumber, seeded and cut into strips
- miso sesame dressing or fish sauce vinaigrette, to dip
- 1 tablespoon toasted sesame seeds
- 1 tablespoon white miso
- 1 tablespoon rice vinegar
- 1 tablespoon kewpie mayo
- pinch of sugar

STEPS

Take a rice paper wrapper and completely submerge it in a bowl of hot tap water for 10-15 seconds. Place the wrapper on a plate or cutting board – it'll continue to soften as your assembling your roll. Add fillings as desired: avocado, smoked salmon, cucumbers, sprouts or noodles. Fold the bottom half of the wrapper up over the filling, hold the fold in place, fold in the sides and roll. Repeat as needed. Dip in the miso sesame dressing or fish sauce vinaigrette and enjoy!

Use a mortar and pestle to crush the sesame seeds. Stir everything together, taste and adjust as needed.

Grab-and-Go Snack Jars

Ingredients

- 1 yellow bell pepper
- 1 red bell pepper
- ½ cup hummus
- ½ cup guacamole
- ½ cup grape tomatoes
- Handful snapea crisps
- ½ cup strawberries
- ½ cup plain Greek yogurt
- ½ cup granola
- ¼ cup blueberries
- ½ cup peanut butter
- 2 celery stalks
- ½ cup pretzels
- Pint mason jars with lids

STEPS

Prepare first jar of bell peppers and hummus. Slice peppers into 1/4-inch strips. Use a spoon to layer in hummus, then top with slices of bell peppers. Seal and store in refrigerator.

Prepare jar of guacamole and black bean crisps. Layer in guacamole first, add in tomatoes for the middle layer, then top with Harvest Snaps black bean habanero crisps. Seal and store in refrigerator. (You want to eat this snack within 24 hours so the crisps don't get soggy.)

Prepare parfait jar. Slice strawberries. Layer in yogurt, granola, strawberries, and blueberries. Seal and store in refrigerator.

Prepare peanut butter and celery jar. Cut celery stalks into 3-inch slices. Layer peanut butter at the bottom, add in celery stick, and top with pretzels. Seal and store in refrigerator. (You also want to eat this snack within 24-48 hours so the pretzels don't get soggy.)

Grab your snacks as needed, whether you're on the go or need an afternoon bite to eat. Enjoy!

Blueberry Coconut Energy Bites

Ingredients

- 1 cup old-fashioned rolled oats (or gluten-free oats)
- ¼ cup ground flaxseed meal
- 2 tablespoons chia seeds
- ¼ teaspoon ground cinnamon
- A pinch of sea salt
- ½ cup creamy almond butter
- ¼ cup honey
- ½ teaspoon vanilla extract
- ½ teaspoon coconut extract, optional
- ¼ cup dried blueberries
- ¼ cup sweetened flaked coconut

STEPS

In a large bowl, combine oats, ground flaxseed, chia seeds, cinnamon, and salt. Place the almond butter in a small microwave safe bowl. Heat in the microwave for 20-30 seconds or until slightly melted. Stir until smooth.

Add the honey, vanilla, and coconut extract, if using, to the melted almond butter. Stir until smooth. Pour over the oat mixture and stir until well combined. Stir in the dried blueberries and coconut.

Roll the mixture into small balls, about 1-2 tablespoons per ball. Place in an airtight container and keep refrigerated for up to 2 weeks. You can also keep the balls in the freezer for up to 1 month.

All-Green Crudités Basket

Ingredients
- 8 ounces/220g string beans or haricot verts, ends trimmed
- 1 head broccoli, cut into florets
- 1 medium cucumber, cut into sticks
- 1 bulb fennel, sliced into thin vertical slices
- 1 bunch celery, cut into sticks
- 1 green pepper, cored, seeded and sliced
- 3 heads endive, large leaves cut in half vertically

STEPS

Bring a large pot of salted water to a boil and fill a large bowl with ice water. Plunge the green beans and broccoli florets into the water and cook until bright green, about 1 minute. Drain and transfer to the ice water bath and let cool completely. Dry on paper towels.

You can use a basket, a bowl, or a box to arrange and present the vegetables. You can also lay them out on a platter. Just group them in large or small clusters, and nestle them closely to one another so that they remain upright.

Falafel Smash

Ingredients
- 1 $\frac{1}{2}$ cups cooked chickpeas drained and rinsed
- $\frac{1}{4}$ teaspoon salt
- 1 teaspoon ground cumin
- 1 teaspoon ground coriander
- $\frac{1}{4}$ teaspoon crushed red pepper
- Juice of $\frac{1}{2}$ lemon
- 1 tablespoon OLIVE OIL
- $\frac{1}{4}$ cup plain non-dairy yogurt
- A few handfuls pea shoots or arugula
- A few slices of pickled red onion thinly sliced raw red onion, or other pickled vegetables
- 4-6 homemade or store-bought pita breads

For the cilantro sauce:
- 1 garlic clove crushed or minced
- 2 large handfuls cilantro finely chopped (including stems)
- $\frac{1}{4}$ cup OLIVE OIL
- 2 tablespoons toasted sesame seeds
- Generous pinch salt

STEPS

In a bowl, lightly mash the chickpeas with the back of a fork, or pulse them briefly in a food processor or countertop blender if you

have one. Stir in the salt, ground cumin, ground coriander, crushed red pepper, lemon juice, and olive oil.
In a small bowl, stir together all the ingredients for the cilantro sauce.
Layer up the yogurt, the pea shoots or arugula, chickpea mixture, cilantro sauce, and pickled or raw red onion on the breads and serve.

Healthy Lemon Bars

Ingredients

For the crust:
- ¼ cup melted and cooled butter, vegan butter or melted coconut oil
- ¼ cup pure maple syrup
- ¼ teaspoon almond extract
- 1 ½ cups packed fine blanched almond flour (do not use almond meal)
- 2 tablespoons coconut flour
- ¼ teaspoon salt

For the filling:
- Zest from 1 lemon
- 2/3 cup freshly squeezed lemon juice (from about 2-4 lemons)
- ½ cup pure maple syrup
- 4 large eggs
- 1 tablespoon coconut flour, sifted (or sub tapioca flour or arrowroot starch)

To garnish:
- Powdered sugar (sifted)
- Lemon zest

STEPS

Preheat oven to 350 °F / 180 ° C.
Line an 8x8 inch pan with parchment paper. (Do not use a glass pan as it will likely cause the bottom of the crust to burn.)
First make the crust: whisk together the almond flour, coconut flour and salt. Next stir in the butter, pure maple syrup and almond extract. Mix until a dough forms. Press dough evenly into prepared pan with your hands. Bake for 15 minutes.
While your crust bakes, you can make the filling: in a medium bowl, whisk together the lemon zest, lemon juice, pure maple syrup, eggs and sifted coconut flour. You want to whisk really well so that no egg white remain visible.
Once crust is done baking, immediately and slowly pour filling over crust. Do not allow the crust to cool first, this is critical.
Lower your oven temperature to 325 degrees F, place bars immediately in oven and bake the bars for 20-25 minutes or until filling is set and no longer jiggles. Cool completely on a wire rack then refrigerate for at least 4 hours to firm up bars. Once ready to serve, use a sharp knife to cut into 12 bars. I recommend garnishing them with powdered sugar and a little lemon zest before serving. Enjoy!

Beet Hummus

Ingredients
- 4 cups canned chickpeas, drained and rinsed
- ⅓ cup extra-virgin olive oil
- 1 medium beet—cooked, peeled and chopped
- ¼ cup fresh lemon juice

- 3 tablespoons tahini
- 1 garlic clove, smashed
- Kosher salt and freshly ground black pepper
- Pita chips, tortilla chips, crackers or chopped vegetables, as desired for dipping

STEPS

In the bowl of a food processor, combine the chickpeas, olive oil, beet, lemon juice, tahini and garlic.
Puree until smooth; season with salt and pepper.
Serve with your choice of chips, crackers and veggies.

Roasted Veggie Chips

Ingredients

- 4 small golden beets
- 4 small red beets
- 2 small turnips
- 2 medium parsnips
- 1 bunch radishes
- 3 tablespoons extra-virgin olive oil
- $1\frac{1}{2}$ tablespoons salt
- 2 teaspoons freshly ground black pepper
- 3 tablespoons chopped fresh herbs (such as rosemary, sage, and/or thyme)

STEPS

Preheat the oven to 400°F/200°C. Line two baking sheets with parchment paper.
Thinly slice the vegetables to about ⅛ inch thick (as thin as you can). Using a mandoline or the slicing side of a box grater can speed up the process, but a knife works just as well. Toss the veggies into a large bowl with the olive oil (you may want to toss the red beets separately to avoid turning everything pink). Spread them in an even layer onto the prepared baking sheets, making sure they do not overlap too much.
Sprinkle the salt, pepper and herbs evenly over the two baking sheets. Roast the vegetables until golden brown and crisp, 20 to 25 minutes. Cool completely before serving. Store in an airtight container to maintain the crisp texture for up to one week.

Rainbow Heirloom Tomato Bruschetta

Ingredients

- 1 baguette, thinly sliced and toasted
- 3 garlic cloves, halved
- 16 ounces/450g whole-milk ricotta cheese
- Kosher salt and freshly ground black pepper
- ¼ cup basil pesto
- 2 tablespoons olive oil
- 2 tablespoons balsamic vinegar
- 2 tablespoons chopped dill sprigs
- 1 red tomato, halved and thinly sliced
- 1 yellow tomato, halved and thinly sliced
- 1 green tomato, halved and thinly sliced
- 1 pint heirloom cherry tomatoes, sliced
- Fresh basil leaves, for serving

STEPS

Rub the surface of each baguette slice with the garlic cloves. Season the ricotta with salt and pepper and then spread onto the baguette slices.

In a medium bowl, whisk together the pesto, olive oil, balsamic vinegar and dill. Add the tomatoes and gently toss to coat.

Working in color blocks, arrange the tomatoes on the baguette slices; season with salt and pepper. Top with basil leaves.

Fava Bean Guacamole With Root Chips

Ingredients

For the root chips:
- 5 large root vegetables (you can use a mix of golden or red beets, or turnips)
- olive oil
- salt

For the spring pea + fava guacamole:
- 20 english peas, peas removed from pod
- 5-6 fava beans, bean removed from pod and outer skin removed
- 4 ripe avocados
- the juice of $\frac{1}{2}$ a lemon
- a handful of cilantro, chopped
- $\frac{1}{2}$ of a small red onion (about 1/4 cup), finely diced
- a pinch of smoked paprika
- salt + pepper
- a pinch of red pepper flakes (optional)

STEPS

Make the root chips:
Pre-heat the oven to 300°. Line a large baking sheet with a piece of parchment paper.

Slice the roots thinly with a mandolin, but not paper thin, you want them to have a little weight to them. Lay the sliced roots out onto the parchment lined baking sheet. Very lightly brush them with olive oil. Do not add salt at this point, it will draw out the water and make the chips soggy.

Place another piece of parchment on top of the roots and then lay another baking sheet on top. This will help keep the chips flat when they bake.

Bake the chips for about 20 minutes. Pull them out and remove the baking sheet that is on top and place them back in the oven for another 15-20 minutes. Keep an eye on them and pull out any that start to brown on the edges.

When the are done, transfer the chips to a wire rack to cool. They will harden and crisp as they cool.

When they've cooled, finish by seasoning with salt.

While the chips are cooling, prepare the gaucamole.

Place a small pot of water on the stove and bring to a boil. Prepare an ice bath and have it ready next to the boiling water.

Place the peas and favas into the boiling water and cook for 3-4 minutes. When the peas and fava beans are tender, remove using a slotted spoon and place into the ice bath. After about 2 minutes, strain the peas and beans from the ice bath.

Smash the avocado with a fork until it is the consistency you like. Add the lemon juice, cilantro, and red onion, smoked paprika and stir to combine. Add the salt, pepper, and red pepper flakes to taste.

Top with the peas and fava beans, and serve immediately with the root chips.

I recommend making the guacamole fresh, and not keeping it around for too long as it will oxidize. The chips, however, can be made ahead of time and stored in an air tight container.

Roasted Pepper And Eggplant Spread Recipe

Ingredients

- 2 pounds / 900g yellow, red, or orange bell peppers (about 5 to 6)
- 1 small eggplant (about 12 ounces)
- 3 tablespoons extra-virgin olive oil divided
- 3 garlic cloves roughly chopped
- 1 ounce / 30 g fresh chives
- 1 tablespoon freshly squeezed lemon juice
- 1 tablespooon red wine vinegar
- 1 teaspoon unrefined cane sugar
- 1/4 teaspoon crushed red pepper flakes
- kosher salt and Freshly ground black pepper

STEPS

Roast The Eggplant and Peppers: Heat oven to 450°F / 220°C and arrange racks in the upper third. Halve each pepper, discarding stems and seeds. Place peppers, cut side down, on a baking sheet lined with foil.

Cut eggplant in half lengthwise and drizzle it with about 1 tablespoon of the olive oil and a little salt and place it, cut-side down, on the baking sheet. Roast the peppers and eggplant until they are blackened, blistered, and the eggplant collapses when you press on it, about 30 minutes.

Peel The Eggplant and Peppers: Remove the eggplant and set it aside to cool slightly. Remove the peppers, place them in a bowl, and cover with plastic wrap until the peppers have slightly cooled, at least 5 minutes. Use a spoon or ice-cream scoop to remove the pulp of the eggplant from the skin, and discard the skin.

Put eggplant in a food processor with 1 tablespoon of the olive oil and the garlic. Pulse the eggplant a few times so that it's roughly chopped.

Make The Ajvar Dip:

Once peppers are cool enough to handle, peel them (reserving any juices that collect), discard the peel, and add the peppers and 2 to 3 tablespoons of the pepper liquid to the food processor. Add the chives and pulse 5 to 8 times to chop coarsely. Stir in the lemon juice, vinegar, red pepper flakes, and sugar. Taste and add more sugar if it is a bit sour, then add salt and freshly ground black pepper, as desired. Serve warm or room temperature as a spread or condiment.

Baked Popcorn Chicken

Ingredients

- 1 ½ pounds / 680g boneless, skinless chicken thighs, cut into 1-inch chunks
- 2 cups low-fat buttermilk
- 3 cloves garlic, smashed
- 1 teaspoon dried basil
- 1 teaspoon dried oregano
- ½ teaspoon dried thyme

- ¼ teaspoon cayenne pepper, optional
- Kosher salt and freshly ground black pepper, to taste
- 3 cups crushed Sour Cream and Onion Kettle Brand® Potato Chips
- ¼ cup unsalted butter, melted
- 2 tablespoons chopped fresh parsley leaves

STEPS

Preheat oven to 400 ° F/ 200 °C. Coat a cooling rack with nonstick spray and place on a baking sheet; set aside.

In a large bowl, combine chicken, buttermilk, garlic, basil, oregano, thyme, cayenne pepper, salt and pepper, to taste; marinate for at least 30 minutes. Drain well.

Working in batches, dredge chicken in crushed potato chips, pressing to coat. Place onto the prepared baking sheet; drizzle with butter.

Place into oven and bake, turning pieces halfway through, until crisp and cooked through, about 20-25 minutes.

Serve immediately, garnished with parsley, if desired.

Pumpkin Hummus

Ingredients

- Two 15-ounce cans chickpeas
- 4 garlic cloves
- ¼ tablespoon extra-virgin olive oil
- 6 tablespoons tahini
- 4 to 6 tablespoons fresh lemon juice (1 to 2 lemons)
- ½ cup pumpkin purée
- Pumpkin spice, cumin, salt and white pepper, to taste

STEPS

Place chickpeas and one garlic clove in a medium pot over high heat and cover with an inch of water. Bring it to a boil, then reduce the heat to medium-low and simmer the chickpeas undisturbed until they start falling apart, about 20 minutes.

Reserve one cup of cooking liquid, then drain the chickpeas and transfer them to a food processor. Add the remaining garlic, olive oil, tahini, lemon juice, pumpkin purée and two tablespoons of reserved cooking liquid to the food processor. Process for about 5 minutes.

If the hummus appears dry or very thick, add more lemon juice, water and/or olive oil to taste to adjust the consistency. Process again until creamy and smooth. Finish the hummus with desired spices and toppings. Serve immediately.

Triple-Berry Smoothie Bowl

Ingredientes

- 1 frozen banana
- 1 cup blueberries
- 1 cup strawberries
- 1 cup raspberries
- ¼ cup Greek yogurt
- ½ cup ice
- ¼ cup blackberries
- 2 tablespoons pumpkin seeds
- 2 tablespoons granola
- 1 tablespoon flaxseeds

STEPS

In a blender, combine the banana, blueberries, strawberries, raspberries, Greek yogurt and ice; blend until smooth.
Divide the smooth between two bowls; top each with blackberries, pumpkin seeds, granola and flaxseeds.

Vegan Brownie Bites

Ingredients
- 1 cups raw cashews or walnuts
- 4 tablespoons raw cacao or cocoa powder, plus extra for rolling (if desired)
- Generous pinch sea salt
- ½ teaspoon vanilla extract (optional)
- 1 ½ cups pitted, tightly packed Medjool dates

STEPS

Place the cashews, cacao powder, and sea salt in a food processor fitted with the S blade. Process for about 30 seconds, or till everything is pretty well ground up.
Add the dates and process for another 1-2 minutes, or until the mixture is evenly combined and sticking together. It should stick together easily when you squeeze a little in your hand.
Shape the "dough" into balls that are about 3/4 – 1 inch thick by rolling it in your palms. If you'd like, transfer extra cacao or cocoa powder to a plate and roll the balls in it to coat.
Store the energy bites in the fridge for 30 minutes, or until ready to eat. Enjoy!

Crispy BBQ Roasted Chickpeas

Ingredientes
- 1 (15-ounce) can chickpeas (very well drained + thoroughly dried)
- 1 Tbsp avocado or other neutral oil (if avoiding oil, omit and don't rinse chickpeas — just drain)
- 2 tsp maple syrup
- 1 ½ tsp smoked paprika
- 1 tsp chili powder
- ¾ tsp garlic powder
- ¼ tsp sea salt
- ¼ tsp black pepper
- ¼ tsp cayenne pepper (optional

STEPS

Preheat oven to 350 º F (180 º C) and set out a bare (or parchment-lined) baking sheet (or more as needed).
Drain chickpeas well. If using oil, rinse well with water and thoroughly drain. If omitting oil, simply drain well and skip rinsing with water.
Once drained well, spread the chickpeas out on a clean, absorbent towel and use your hands to gently roll and dry the chickpeas. Some of the skins should start coming off. You can opt to peel all of the chickpeas — which can help for extra crispiness! — or simply remove the skins that come off. Either way, the chickpeas will crisp up. I just found that peeling them does yield slightly crispier chickpeas.
Transfer the chickpeas to a mixing bowl and top with oil. Mix well to combine. DO NOT add the other seasonings at this point —

they can interrupt the crisping process, so wait to add until after baking.

Bake for 45 minutes or until golden brown and dry/crispy to the touch. We like turning the pan around and shaking the chickpeas around the halfway point for even cooking. Note: Peeled chickpeas cook faster than unpeeled. If omitting oil, they will also cook faster.

Remove your chickpeas from the oven and prepare your BBQ seasoning. In a medium-size mixing bowl, combine the maple syrup, smoked paprika, chili powder, garlic powder, sea salt, black pepper, and cayenne (optional) until a paste forms.

Pour in your still-warm chickpeas and toss gently to evenly coat them with the seasoning mixture. Place them back on the cookie sheet to cool fully and so the seasoning can dry/set.

Enjoy as a protein-rich snack or use atop things like grain bowls, kale salads, or our easy and summery chopped salad! To store, place in a storage container or jar and DO NOT tightly cover. Instead, crack lid so they can "breathe" a bit. This helps them stay crispy longer. These are best the first day, but they will last for 4-5 days at room temperature. Alternatively, seal well and freeze up to 1 month.

Veggie Sushi

Ingredients

Rice
- 1½ cups sushi rice
- 1¾ cups water
- 3 tablespoons rice vinegar
- 1 tablespoon sugar
- 1¼ teaspoons salt

Sushi
- 2 European cucumbers
- 1½ cups thinly sliced carrots (½-inch pieces)
- 1 avocado, pitted and thinly sliced into ½-inch pieces
- ½ bunch scallions, cut into ½-inch pieces
- Soy sauce, for dipping

STEPS

MAKE THE RICE:
In a medium pot, combine the rice with the water. Bring the mixture to a boil over medium heat. Reduce the heat to low, cover the pot and let simmer until the rice absorbs all the water and is tender, 9 to 10 minutes. In a small pot, bring the rice vinegar to a simmer over medium-low heat. Stir in the sugar and salt until they're fully dissolved. Pour the vinegar mixture
over the rice and use a spatula to toss the rice to coat.
Cool completely.

MAKE THE SUSHI:
Cut the ends off the cucumbers and then thinly slice the cucumbers into long ⅛-inch-thick strips.
Dip your hands into cool water and then mound 1 rounded tablespoon of rice and press it firmly into a tight ball.
Place the rice ball at one end of a cucumber strip. Place a few pieces of carrot,
a piece of avocado and a piece of scallion alongside the rice.

Roll up the ingredients to wrap fully in the cucumber. Secure the end of the cucumber with a toothpick. Repeat with the remaining rice, cucumber strips and veggies. You can remove the toothpicks after the rolls have set for 5 minutes. Transfer to a serving platter.

Serve immediately with soy sauce.

Conclusions

The Mediterranean diet consists of a lifestyle based on a balanced and varied diet in which foods obtained from the traditional crops of this geographical area bathed by the Mediterranean predominate: wheat, olive trees, and grapes.

Epidemiological and clinical studies support the benefits of this diet. In vitro research conducted in the laboratory shows that consuming these foods decreases oxidative stress and is preventive for obesity, Alzheimer's disease, diabetes, arterial hypertension, cancer, osteoporosis, cardiovascular diseases, and premature deaths derived from these pathologies.

The benefits of this diet are:

- Low contribution in saturated fats.
- High contribution in monounsaturated fats.
- Balanced in polyunsaturated fatty acids (omega-3 and omega-6).
- Low intake of animal protein.
- Rich in antioxidants.
- Rich in fiber.
- Rich in complex carbohydrates.
- Its positive health effects

Among the beneficial effects of the Mediterranean diet for our health, we highlight:

- Decrease in total cholesterol and LDL (low intensity).
- Increased HDL cholesterol (beneficial for health).
- Increased antioxidant capacity of the body.
- It raises vitamin C, E, beta-carotene, and polyphenols in the blood.
- It lowers blood pressure levels because it has little sodium and is abundant in potassium and fiber.
- Helps detoxify substances in the liver.
- Reduces the risk of thrombosis, acting on the coagulation mechanisms.
- It protects the arteries, dilating them and stimulating the production of the enzyme nitric oxide sin to erase from the endothelium (inner layer of the arteries).
- Reduces inflammatory reactions.
- It modifies the expression of genes, making them healthier and increasing the immune defense capacity.

In short, the Mediterranean diet as a reference diet has a beneficial effect on health. Within the Mediterranean diet, it is difficult to determine the beneficial effect attributable to olive oil rich in oleic acid and vitamin E or that attributable to other foods such as fish, cereals, or legumes. Therefore, the Mediterranean diet should be considered a whole, in which the beneficial effects of the different components are surely additive or synergistic. Since several substances have beneficial effects present in different foods in varying amounts, today, almost all food guides emphasize the importance of consuming a very varied diet that incorporates many unprocessed foods such as fresh fruits and vegetables.

Likewise, when judging the positive effects of the Mediterranean diet, we must not forget the role that other non-dietary factors related to the culture of the Mediterranean regions possibly play in the low incidence of chronic diseases, such as calmer life stress, nap, etc.

The Mediterranean eating style has shown, with broad scientific solvency, by association or intervention, to generate numerous benefits in preventing and treating different risk conditions and chronic pathologies. There are five Mediterranean ecosystems globally, and their local agricultural and aquaculture production is very abundant in products associated with the Mediterranean diet. In addition, some studies indicate that the benefits of the Mediterranean diet are replicable in countries outside the Mediterranean basin. All the evidence reviewed suggests that the Mediterranean-type diet is an important tool to be implemented at the public health level in developing effective policies to reduce premature morbidity and mortality in the population.

Numerous studies have linked the Mediterranean diet with a better state of health, reducing mortality, incidence of cancer, cardiovascular and neurodegenerative diseases. Many of these studies have analyzed specific foods (such as olive oil) or some of their compounds. Still, the evidence indicates that the combination of them and their interaction enhances the state of health.

Studies carried out on the effects produced by the main foods of the Mediterranean diet on the human body show the following results:

– Olive oil contains:

Vitamins A (growth and development, good vision, immune system), D (calcium absorption, bone mineralization), E (lipid antioxidant, antiatherogenic, prevents arteriosclerosis), and K (blood coagulation).
Polyphenols, whose antioxidant action slows down cell aging and hinders the formation of cancer cells.
Oleic acid reduces LDL cholesterol, triglycerides, high blood pressure, and insulin resistance. In addition, it increases the body's defenses, reduces the risk of rheumatoid arthritis and gastric acidity, prevents peptic ulcers, and regulates gastric motility.

– Fruits and vegetables provide a large amount of water and, among other components, dietary fiber, vitamins C, A, E, and K, folic acid, beta-carotene and other carotenoids, polyphenols, phytoestrogens, tocopherols, minerals (magnesium, potassium, sodium, calcium, iron…), etc.

The daily intake of this food group reduces the risk of cardiovascular and neurodegenerative diseases, depression, neural tube defects, and some types of cancer (lung, digestive system, prostate, breast...); prevents constipation and high blood pressure; improves the condition of the skin, hair, nails, and teeth, as well as mood, quality of sleep and blood circulation; protects eye health, reduces insulin resistance, helps eliminate uric acid and toxins, and benefits the nervous and immune systems.

Its high fiber content has a satiating effect and low-calorie content, helping maintain a healthy weight. Many vitamins and minerals have antioxidant effects, which play a key role in reducing disease and slowing aging.

Nuts contain mono and polyunsaturated fatty acids, arginine, folic and alpha-linolenic acids, vitamin E, minerals (magnesium, potassium, phosphorus, selenium…), phytosterols, and other bioactive components, which exert a protective action against disease coronary due to its hypocholesterolemic effect.

Cereals are mainly made up of carbohydrates, such as starch. They contain small amounts of protein and lipids. They also provide mineral salts, some B vitamins, and fiber, but they are lost if subjected to a refining process. There is some evidence that supports the consumption of whole grains for their beneficial effects in preventing cardiovascular diseases, type 2 diabetes, and certain cancers of the digestive system.

Legumes are a source of very good quality protein, close to those of animal origin. Carbohydrates, especially in the form of starch, are its main macronutrient, followed by raffinose and stachyose. They are high in soluble and insoluble fiber, vitamins B1, B3, and B6, folate, minerals (calcium, phosphorus, potassium, magnesium, iron, and zinc), and other components of nutritional interest (phenolic compounds, phytoestrogens, condensed tannins, etc.), as well as some less desirable ones (oligosaccharides, phytic acid, and enzyme inhibitors). They prevent type 2 diabetes, hypertension, cancer, hypercholesterolemia, and inflammatory diseases.

Fish have an excellent nutritional value, similar to that of meat. They provide between 15-24% of proteins of high biological value since they contain all the essential amino acids in the optimal amount for the body. They provide a wide variety of vitamins (thiamin, riboflavin, retinol, calciferol, tocopherol, etc.) and minerals (phosphorus, potassium, magnesium, calcium, selenium, iron, zinc, iodine…). Fish fat is rich in polyunsaturated fatty acids, especially omega-3 (more abundant in oily fish). These fatty acids can reduce high blood pressure, triglycerides, blood clotting, the risk of heart failure and stroke.

Eggs have a complete nutritional value, as they contain all the essential amino acids. They provide carotenoids, vitamins such as A, D and E, several from group B (cobalamin, folic acid, choline, riboflavin), and iron, calcium, and phosphorus magnesium. Its protein, ovalbumin, is of the highest quality; It is found in the white of the egg and represents almost 60% of the total weight. Its fatty acids are 2/3 mono and polyunsaturated (mainly alpha-linoleic omega 3) and 1/3 saturated. Due to its excellent nutritional quality and its numerous bioactive compounds, the egg is a recommended food for people with higher nutritional demand, such as children, the elderly, or pregnant women. However, it is recommended to restrict its consumption (or avoid the yolk) in the diabetic or high cardiovascular risk population.

Meats make a great contribution to proteins of high biological value since, of their amino acids, approximately 40% are essential. The fat content varies depending on the species and part of the animal; about 50% are saturated fats. They provide few carbohydrates (normally in the form of glycogen) and very little fiber. They are a considerable source of iron and other minerals (zinc, magnesium, phosphorus, selenium, copper...). Usually, They contain B vitamins (B1, B3, B5, B6, B12, and biotin), vitamin A (retinol), vitamin E, and folic acid (lamb and sheep). Moderate consumption of meat is recommended, especially red and processed, because, although they are important for muscle formation and recovery after exertion, it is considered that they may be related to cardiovascular diseases and various types of cancer.

Dairy products provide high biological value (casein and whey proteins) and contain all the essential amino acids in human nutrition. They provide vitamins A, D, E, K, several of the B group, and minerals (especially calcium, and, to a lesser extent, phosphorus, potassium, magnesium, zinc, and others). The main carbohydrate is lactose, which facilitates calcium absorption, although digestive intolerance can cause it. They contain cholesterol and a predominance of saturated fatty acids (60-70%) compared to unsaturated ones. Milk consumption promotes bone development and the formation of new tissues in the body, prevents osteoporosis, has a uricosuric effect, neutralizes stomach acid, and promotes microbiota growth.

Moderate alcohol intake (10 to 30 g of ethanol per day), especially red wine, is one of the characteristics of the Mediterranean diet. Many studies show that this habit reduces cardiovascular mortality due to its effect on plasmatic lipoproteins (it raises HDL cholesterol and reduces, although less, LDL cholesterol). In addition, it decreases platelet aggregability and causes changes in fibrinolysis and coagulation. There is insufficient evidence on the antioxidant role of its polyphenols, nor on a beneficial effect of any other component other than ethanol.

Even though there is some controversy regarding the quality of the studies, the Mediterranean diet enjoys considerable acceptance, being considered a model of a prudent and healthy diet.

Manufactured by Amazon.ca
Bolton, ON

27600604R00072